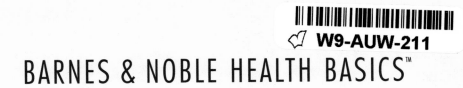

BARNES & NOBLE HEALTH BASICS™

Diabetes

by Paul Heltzel

BARNES
&NOBLE
BOOKS
NEW YORK

About the Author

Paul Heltzel was diagnosed with type 1 diabetes when he was 10 years old and has lived with the disease in good health for 23 years. He is a science and technology reporter and teaches journalism at Tulane's University College, where he serves as an adjunct faculty member in the Media Arts department. This is his eighth book.

About the Contributors

Portions of this work were reviewed by Stephen Possick, M.D. , and Marcy Adlersberg Cheifetz, M.D., Clinical Instructor, Yale University, and Clinical Endocrinologist, Waterbury Hospital, Waterbury, CT. The nutritional information was written by Mindy Hermann, R.D. The information about complementary therapies was written by Melanie Hulse.

Barbara J. Morgan Publisher, Silver Lining Books
Barnes & Noble Basics

Barb Chintz Editorial Director
Barbara Rietschel Art Director
Clellen Bryant Editor
Emily Seese Editorial Assistant
Della R. Mancuso Production Manager

Illustrations by Cynthia Saniewski

Table of Contents

Foreword

If you or a loved one has just received a diagnosis of diabetes, the first thing you will want to do is to learn about it so you can manage the condition effectively. This is where Barnes & Noble Health Basics *Diabetes* comes in. Written with expert guidance from leading physicians, this informative book leads you to a deeper understanding of your symptoms and treatment.

No matter what type of diabetes you have, you'll find plenty of useful information on treatment, medication, nutrition, complementary therapies, searching the Internet, and putting together a health-care team. You'll also get the latest news on cutting-edge research and some wise advice on the role of stress and comfort in managing your health.

With all of these helpful insights at your fingertips, you'll be able to take control of your diabetes and become an advocate for your own health care. Remember: An informed patient is an empowered one. So read on to put yourself in the driver's seat when it comes to treating and managing your diabetes.

Barb Chintz
Editorial Director
Barnes & Noble Health Basics Series

CHAPTER 1

Getting the Diagnosis

Experiencing the symptoms
subtle signals from your body

What does it feel like to have diabetes? Sometimes it feels like nothing out of the ordinary. About one third of those who have diabetes don't even know it. The symptoms can be so subtle that many people just carry on with their lives or dismiss them as symptoms of stress—that is, until the symptoms worsen to the point where a visit to the doctor is in order. It's possible that you had no inkling that you had diabetes until you had a routine blood test at your regular physical examination.

Or you may have suffered one or more of the classic symptoms of diabetes. Maybe you felt drowsy or had to urinate more frequently than usual, getting up often at night to do so. You might have been unusually thirsty or hungry. Perhaps you lost weight for no apparent reason, something that is welcome to many people and therefore not likely to cause concern. More worrisome, maybe you had an occasional episode of blurry vision. Or you felt some tingling or numbness or even pain in your legs and feet. Perhaps you got more infections than usual, and cuts healed more slowly than they used to.

You probably didn't have all of these symptoms, just one or two. And it's possible, though highly unlikely, that your doctor didn't piece your symptoms together and sent you on your way with a warning to regulate your weight. The reason for a missed diagnosis is twofold. Most people don't pay the right kind of attention to their bodies and they don't know how to talk effectively to their doctors about their symptoms. Whenever a doctor and a patient talk, there are bound to be miscommunications. Think back to the time your car was on the fritz. Remember how you tried to explain the clunk-clunk noise to your mechanic and how he looked at you quizzically? Well, talking to your doctor about your symptoms can be just as difficult sometimes. (For more on how to overcome this natural communication problem, see page 78.)

Even those who are in tune with their bodies are amazed at how subtle some diabetes symptoms can be. What can you do about this communication gap? For starters, you need to know the symptoms that arise with diabetes. They fall into two main groups. One group of symptoms is caused by type 1 diabetes, and the other is due to type 2 diabetes. Having several of these symptoms does not mean that you have diabetes, but it does mean that you need to talk to your doctor about them. Below is a roundup of typical diabetes symptoms.

Common Symptoms of Diabetes

Type 1 Diabetes (symptoms come on quickly)	**Type 2 Diabetes** (symptoms come on slowly)
Excessive hunger with no weight gain	Increased urination
Excessive thirst	Fatigue
Unexplained weight loss	Increased thirst
Frequent urination, often at night	Blurred vision
Fatigue and drowsiness	More frequent infections
Nausea and vomiting	Sores that don't heal
Fruity breath odor	Numbness or tingling in the feet or legs
Rapid breathing	Dry, itchy skin

Seeing your doctor
what your doctor looks for

Regardless of whether your symptoms come on suddenly or gradually, there usually comes a point when they become so pronounced that you see your doctor. If your doctor suspects diabetes, then the very first thing he or she will do is order a **morning fasting glucose test**. This test is taken in the morning on an empty stomach. The goal is to measure your blood glucose level while it is at its lowest point in the day.

Why all this concern with **glucose**? Because whenever you take a bite of food or a sip of a drink, a very delicate metabolic dance begins. Here's how it starts: Substances in your food and drink are first broken down into various chemicals that your body can use, namely protein, fat and cholesterol, and sugar (also known as glucose). Protein is then processed and put to use to build muscles, skin, hair, and blood, among other things. Fat is processed and used to cushion the organs, among other things. Sugar (glucose) is absorbed into the bloodstream, where it moves into various cells of the body to be used or stored for later. Glucose cannot automatically be absorbed into your bloodstream; it needs a special chemical transport to get there. Enter **insulin,** a hormone made by the **pancreas**—the banana-shaped gland that sits behind your stomach. When the body senses the presence of glucose in the blood, the pancreas releases insulin, which moves the glucose into the body's cells or stores it for future use.

This fine balancing act is known as an **endocrine feedback loop.** It's this constant feedback between the pancreas and the presence of blood sugar that keeps all your cells properly energized. But sometimes there are problems with this delicate loop. Either there is not enough insulin, or there is enough insulin but your body has built up a resistance to it. If there is not enough insulin to move glucose from the blood into the body's cells, then glucose remains in the blood. When the blood glucose levels become too high, the glucose spills over into the urine. When the glucose levels in the urine get too high, the kidneys produce excess urine. This leads to frequent urination and excessive thirst. The cycle builds, resulting in dehydration, dizziness, fatigue, blurred vision, and a host of other symptoms. The bottom line? Diabetes mellitus. (*Mellitus* is Latin for "honey" or, in this case, "sugar." *Dia* is Greek for "through" and *betes* is Greek for "flowing." Put them together and you have "sugar flowing through"; in other words, sugar flowing through the kidneys and into the urine.)

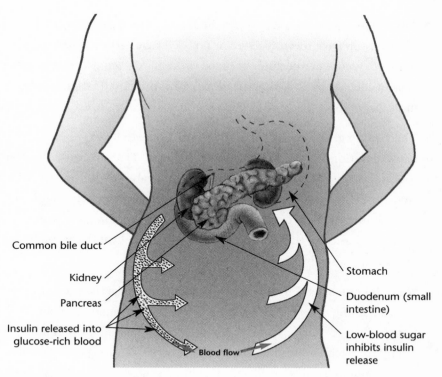

Common bile duct

Kidney

Pancreas

Insulin released into
glucose-rich blood

Blood flow

Stomach

Duodenum (small
intestine)

Low-blood sugar
inhibits insulin
release

The constant feedback between the pancreas (shown here in blue) and the level of blood sugar keeps your body's cells energized. Here is how it works: When food is eaten, the pancreas releases insulin into the blood so the sugar in food can enter the cells of the body as glucose. Simultaneously, the muscle and liver cells convert glucose to glycogen. When there is no presence of food (or low blood sugar), insulin release is inhibited.

Tests for diabetes
what your doctor tests

If your doctor suspects diabetes, then he or she will order various blood tests to track the amount of glucose in your blood. Remember that glucose gets into our bodies when we digest certain types of foods. Because diabetes involves moving glucose from the blood into the body's cells, doctors can use blood tests to determine your glucose levels. There are three basic blood tests doctors use:

◆ **The blood glucose test** can be taken at any time, regardless of whether you have recently eaten or not. A level of 200 milligrams or more of glucose per deciliter of blood (200 mg/dl) along with the presence of such diabetic symptoms as excessive thirst and fatigue, is an indicator of diabetes.

◆ **The fasting glucose test** For eight hours before this test, you are allowed nothing to eat and only water to drink. That's because this test is designed to measure your blood sugar at its absolute lowest level, well after you have digested your last meal. A reading of 110 mg/dl or lower indicates that you do not have diabetes. A reading of 126 mg/dl or higher indicates that you have diabetes, especially if these results are accompanied by diabetic symptoms.

◆ **The oral glucose tolerance test** This test begins like the previous one, with a reading of your blood sugar after you have fasted for eight hours. Then you are asked to drink a very sweet liquid on your still-empty stomach and wait for another two hours. At that point, you are tested again to see how well your insulin has handled the shot of sweet liquid and subsequent sharp rise in blood sugar. If your blood sugar reading is 200 mg/dl or higher, your doctor will definitely tell you that you have diabetes. (This test is used in Europe and most other countries to diagnose diabetes.)

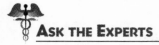

Ask the Experts

Is there any way I could get a false reading?

No laboratory is 100 percent accurate. False positives do occur. That's why a blood glucose reading of over 200 mg/dl needs to be accompanied by symptoms to be meaningful. For final confirmation, your doctor will usually ask you to take two fasting glucose tests, to be given on two separate mornings.

My glucose levels came back "borderline" for diabetes. What does that mean?

This is not that uncommon. If your levels are between 110 and 125 mg/dl, you may be diagnosed with something called **impaired glucose tolerance**, or IGT. Those who have IGT are considered at risk of developing full-blown diabetes down the road. The good news is that with proper diet and exercise and close monitoring by your doctor, you can prevent diabetes from developing. Studies have shown a 60 percent reduction in risk of developing diabetes in patients with IGT who diet and exercise. People with IGT also need to watch their cholesterol level and blood pressure, because those with any risk of diabetes are also at risk of developing heart disease (see pages 146–147 for more information).

Types of diabetes
there are three kinds

How your diabetes starts and how your doctor treats it depend on the type of diabetes you have. There are three main types of diabetes. All three reflect the same problem: the body's inability to process the sugars and starches we eat into the fuel that our bodies use for energy.

◆ **Type 1 diabetes** Here, the pancreas no longer makes insulin. Type 1 diabetes is an autoimmune disease that most often occurs in people under the age of 30 and that was formerly referred to as juvenile diabetes. About 10 percent of people with diabetes have type 1.

◆ **Type 2 diabetes** The pancreas produces too little insulin or the body is resistant to the insulin it does produce and cannot use it effectively. Type 2 diabetes used to be called adult-onset diabetes. Type 2 diabetes can sometimes be prevented or delayed by eating a healthy diet, exercising, and losing weight.

◆ **Gestational diabetes** About 3 to 6 percent of all pregnant women get this temporary syndrome, which starts when pregnancy hormones cause resistance to insulin, elevating blood sugar levels. With diet, many women with gestational diabetes can control their glucose levels, but some need to take insulin. After the baby is born, gestational diabetes usually goes away, but sometimes it doesn't, and then it becomes a case of type 2 diabetes and is treated accordingly. (A woman with diabetes who becomes pregnant will need to work with her doctor to adjust her insulin levels to deal with the increased blood sugar that occurs during pregnancy.)

How Did Diabetes Start?

No one is certain, but there are some intriguing theories that try to offer partial explanations. One is that ancient populations that endured frequent cycles of feast and famine developed a different kind of metabolism than those with reliable food supplies as a way of coping with starvation, and their descendants have more difficulty adapting to a world where there is plenty to eat. Type 2 diabetes is more prevalent among African-Americans, Hispanics, Asian-Americans, Pacific Islanders, and Native Americans. The latter in particular often have problems with weight, and in some groups half the adults have type 2 diabetes. On the other hand, type 1 diabetes is rarer among those groups than in the general population and occurs more frequently in people whose ancestors came from cold climates such as northern Europe, especially Scandinavia. There is a theory that type 1 diabetes may be caused by a virus, and viral infections are more common in winter.

Can stress affect your blood sugar?

When your body reacts to stress, you usually experience some very distinct bodily changes. Your heart races to increase blood to the muscles; glucose levels in the blood increase to better fuel your muscles; your breathing increases to get more oxygen to the brain so it stays alert; and your digestion shuts down in order to send energy to the muscles. These are just a few of the responses that are hardwired into your body to help it handle a stressful situation. Once the stress has passed, your body then returns to its normal restful state. But what happens if there are chronic zaps of the stress responses and the body never gets a chance to return to a restful state? The body remains in a constant state of alert. For people with diabetes, that means elevated levels of glucose in the blood. For this health reason and others, it is vital to learn how to manage stress so it does not worsen any existing health problems. For more on stress, see pages 155–170.

Getting a diagnosis
there is a range of emotions

Everyone reacts differently to being told they have diabetes. Some people immediately focus on their treatment. Others are so shocked that they leave the doctor's office without asking a single question. If it's type 2 diabetes, a lot of people feel tremendous guilt because they think their eating habits caused the illness. If they have type 1, they often feel angry at their bodies for "betraying" them. The best way to view this illness is to consider it as just another of life's challenges that you can manage. You are not good or bad for getting this disorder. It simply happened. Sure, being overweight may have been part of the problem, but genetics also plays an important role. Your task now is to learn how to manage your illness and live your life to the fullest. To that end, your first step will be to work out a treatment plan with your doctor or a diabetes educator (see pages 67–82).

Okay, yes, you will likely need to change significant aspects of your lifestyle. And yes, you will have to make changes to your diet. You may have to take pills or injections (or both). The good news is that all these changes require you to be in charge, which is not the case with many diseases. You can learn how to manage this chronic illness. It just takes time and effort. The key is control, and not just the obviously important control of your blood sugar, but emotional control. You can take control through:

- ◆ Forming a two-way partnership with your doctor.

- ◆ Creating a health journal (see pages 22–23).

- ◆ Becoming a proactive patient and involving family, friends, and others in a circle of help (see pages 76–77).

- ◆ Making the most of nonmedicinal treatments, such as exercise and relaxation (see pages 105–118).

- ◆ Finding a way to manage your diabetes that fits your lifestyle (see pages 119–130).

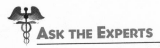

Can't I just carry on with my life?

Yes—and no. Yes, you can have a long life and live it to the fullest, enjoying everything you do or planned to do. But no, you cannot ignore your diabetes, because it is never going to just go away. It will be your constant companion. Now is also the time to take seriously all those good resolutions you have made and broken over the years, and to reap the benefits of doing so. For instance, because exercise is a must for people with diabetes, you will be motivated to get in better shape. The same for losing weight, which can help reduce insulin resistance, improve circulation, and lower blood pressure.

The shock of getting a diagnosis

Everyone reacts differently when they get a diagnosis of a chronic disorder. If your symptoms were nominal, then the common reaction is surprise and an immediate focus on treatment. But for those who have been plagued with uncomfortable symptoms for more than a few weeks or months, there can be a whole host of feelings, from fear and guilt to sadness and anger. Sometimes being told you have a named illness can trigger the stress response. This is when your breathing becomes shallow and blood rushes to your muscles. These physical responses help you cope with a perceived threat, but such an intense physical response sometimes short-circuits your brain, so you think and remember less clearly than normally. This could explain why so many people cannot quite take in what their doctor is saying when they get their diagnosis, let alone what treatment plans they need to follow. Oftentimes, it's only when they get home and relax that the news of the diagnosis can fully sink in.

Possible causes
why me, why now?

The causes behind the three types of diabetes are diverse. But they all revolve around one particular gland, the pancreas. Most people never have reason to give much thought to the gland known as the pancreas. This banana-shaped, fist-size gland sits behind your stomach and produces the enzymes and hormones that help with digestion. How does it do this? Spread throughout the pancreas are bundles of cells called **islets of Langerhans,** about 100,000 of them, named after Paul Langerhans, the German physician who first discovered them in 1869. In the islets, one type of cell, called an **alpha cell,** makes the hormone **glucagon,** which forces cells to release or produce glucose (from ingested carbohydrates), thereby raising blood sugar. But it is another type of islet cell, the **beta cell,** that does most of the heavy lifting. It acts as a sort of meter, responding to the level of glucose in your blood by making and releasing a corresponding amount of the hormone **insulin** to keep your blood sugar level in check. Insulin works by helping the cells absorb glucose, thereby lowering blood sugar. All day, every day, the pancreas continuously balances the two hormones to keep your blood sugar level within a healthy range.

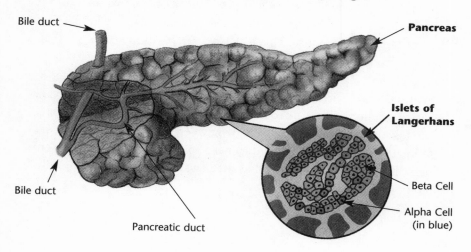

Bile duct

Pancreas

Islets of
Langerhans

Beta Cell

Bile duct

Alpha Cell
(in blue)

Pancreatic duct

In type 1 diabetes, the autoimmune system attacks the beta cells in the islets. Yes, that can sound scary, but actually autoimmune disorders are more common than you realize. Normally, when the body is under attack from a virus or an infection, it issues antibodies to kill off these foreign invaders. In an autoimmune disease, the body gets confused and cannot tell foreign cells from normal cells. The result? The body attacks its own normal cells thinking that it is helping, when, in fact, it is doing much damage. Usually autoimmune disorders target a particular part of the body; for example, in rheumatoid arthritis, the body's joints are attacked. In type 1 diabetes, the beta cells in the pancreas are destroyed, so insulin cannot be produced.

The causes of type 2 diabetes are less well known and more complex, though researchers have determined that obesity can trigger type 2 diabetes. If you have type 2 diabetes, your pancreas may produce plenty of insulin. In fact, it may overproduce insulin, but your body is unable to use the insulin that the pancreas delivers because it has become insulin-resistant. Alternatively, some individuals with type 2 diabetes may have fewer than the normal number of beta cells and so produce too little insulin. Or there may be problems with the mechanism that determines whether blood sugar is high or low and calls for more or less production of insulin.

You are not alone
welcome to a very large club

Once you have been diagnosed with diabetes, you will suddenly become aware of how many people you know who have diabetes and how many other people there are in the world with diabetes. One of the first things you will notice is the number of famous people who have diabetes. For instance, Halle Berry has diabetes, and so does George Lucas, Mary Tyler Moore, and Elizabeth Taylor. So, for that matter, did Jackie Robinson, Thomas Edison, and Nikita Khrushchev. The list is endless. The point is that diabetes didn't keep any of those people down, and there is no reason it should hold you back, either.

About 17 million people in the United States have diabetes (90 percent have type 2 diabetes), so whether you know it or not, you will have lots of company wherever you go. Diabetes is one of the most studied of diseases, and the care of it is thoroughly organized. There are plenty of people out there who have gone through what you are going through, and plenty of people who are waiting to help you. In the front ranks are your physician, who will help map out your plan for handling your diet and medication, and your diabetes educator (see page 72), who will guide you through the management of the disease.

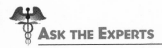

How close is a cure for diabetes? Will I have diabetes for the rest of my life?

It's impossible to say. While the problem seems simple (you need insulin for energy), a cure is complicated. That's because type 1 and type 2 diabetes are dramatically different diseases, so one cure would not fit all. Fortunately, there have been a number of breakthroughs in diabetic research and treatment over the past 20 years. Until a cure is found, you need to watch your diabetes carefully, see your doctor often, and try to reduce stress. You are doing the very best you can.

FIRST PERSON INSIGHTS

The shocking news

I couldn't believe what my doctor was telling me. I am a 58-year-old high school math teacher with no symptoms or family history of any illnesses. Two days after my annual physical, my doctor telephoned me. My blood and urine tests showed a high glucose concentration, indicating that I probably had diabetes. My immediate reaction was disbelief, then fear. There had been no known history of diabetes in my family. More tests were arranged. On the day my blood was tested for glucose content (after I had fasted for eight hours), it turned out to be higher than normal. I then had to go out and eat a heavy breakfast—bacon, eggs, and pancakes with syrup—before another round of blood tests a couple of hours later. The next day, my GP telephoned again to say that I indeed had type 2 diabetes and that I needed to see him that day to get a prescription for an oral medication. He prescribed two tablets per day. It took a few days, but I finally absorbed my news. I had type 2 diabetes.

—John D., Mission, WY

Keeping a health journal
starting a glucose log

One of the best ways to keep tabs on your health after you have been diagnosed with diabetes is to keep a **glucose log**. Depending on your treatment, you will probably need to check your blood sugar levels at least two times a day, if not more. This is not optional. It involves measuring your blood glucose levels using a very small sample of blood taken from your finger by one of the simple home monitors available today, then jotting down your findings in your glucose log, a small notebook that you carry with you, along with your testing equipment. Most home monitors come with one to help get you started.

Keeping a glucose log will help you learn to pay attention to your body and understand what it is trying to tell you. While you are writing down your glucose readings, it is also vital to keep track of your medicine and diet and exercise. Every day, you will need to make a note of your daily medicine, food intake, and time spent exercising. And, if possible, keep notes on any symptom flare-ups. In doing this, you will be creating a valuable diagnostic tool that will help both you and your doctor, as well as the rest of your support team (see pages 67–82), recognize any patterns of symptoms that may be giving you trouble. And, finally, this log does a wonderful job of reminding you that you, not your doctors, are in charge of your health.

To help organize your files, it is a good idea to create a health journal. Get a three-ring binder with loose-leaf paper and insert several dividers that you can label. You'll need labels for sections, such as General Health, Doctor Visits, Lab Tests, Diet, and the all-important section on Daily Glucose Readings. This section will include past records of your blood sugar readings, pulled from your glucose log.

Glucose Log

Your glucose log needs to be small and portable. You can create your own forms (see below) or download spreadsheet forms from the computer. Check out this site for glucose log forms: **www.mendosa.com/software.htm.** It also describes and reviews current software programs that help you track your glucose levels and manage your diet and exercise program.

	SUN	MON	TUES	WED	THURS	FRI	SAT
GLUCOSE READING							
Before Breakfast							
After Breakfast							
Before Lunch							
Afternoon							
Before Dinner							
After Dinner							
Before Bed							

Helpful resources

The Chronic Illness Workbook
by Patricia Fennel

The American Diabetes Association
A nonprofit organization that promotes education, advocacy, and research. The ADA's *Diabetes Forecast* is a monthly magazine that offers tips for management and articles on research.
www.diabetes.org

The Insulin-Free World Foundation is a cure-focused organization that promotes research on islet and pancreas transplants and works to create a community of diabetics who have received, or want more information about, transplants. The IFW's Web site also offers handy information on insulin-pump therapy.
www.insulinfree.org

The Juvenile Diabetes Research Foundation
A nonprofit organization like the ADA, the JDRF provides information and advice for people with type 1 diabetes. The organization raises money, funds research, and lobbies for legislation that benefits people with diabetes. Mary Tyler Moore (diagnosed with type 1 at age 30) has long been the JDRF's chairperson. The JDRF puts out a monthly magazine, *Countdown*, that accompanies membership.
www.jdrf.org

Treatments

Doing the work of the pancreas
treatment to mimic the pancreas

There was a time when your biggest concern about sugar was one lump or two. But now that you have been diagnosed with diabetes, much of your treatment will revolve around the amount of sugar you consume. It's not just table sugar you will be watching, as your doctor or diabetes educator (see page 72) will tell you, but all the carbohydrates you eat—starches, sugars, vegetables, fruits, and even dairy products contain carbohydrates. In your body, carbohydrates are converted to glucose and then absorbed into the bloodstream thanks to the pancreas's release of insulin. But when you have diabetes, this glucose-insulin loop is not working and your pancreas does not produce enough insulin to absorb the glucose effectively, or your body is resisting the insulin it does supply. That's where treatment comes in. Its job is to mimic the work of the pancreas. Here is a brief overview of what you must do to manage your diabetes:

◆ Keep fairly constant tabs on the amount of glucose in your blood. This calls for measuring your blood for glucose at various intervals throughout the day. There are a number of glucose meters (see pages 28–29) out there to help you keep track of your blood glucose.

◆ Analyze the results of your tests. Do they fall within the normal range for blood glucose? Your doctor will tell you what your particular blood sugar level should be before and after meals, but here are some sample ranges to give you an idea:

Before breakfast	90 to 130
Before lunch, supper, and snack	90 to 130
Two hours after meals	Less than 160
Bedtime	110 to 150

◆ Watch what you eat. Before diabetes, you could pretty much eat what you wanted and your pancreas would sense the presence of sugar in your blood and release insulin to metabolize it. Now, you'll need to monitor the amount of carbohydrates you eat in order to match it to the amount of insulin you will need to process it properly. Food can still be a joy, but it is also a part of your medical treatment.

◆ Take your medication. Depending on which type of diabetes you have, you may need to take pills or give yourself synthetic insulin by injection. For those who need to have insulin injections, know that it will take some time to learn how to manage your insulin intake. Too little insulin and you will have too much sugar in your blood and feel tired and lethargic. Too much insulin and you can develop **hypoglycemia**, a condition of low blood sugar, which can cause shaking, sweating, and anxiety. Severe hypoglycemia can cause confusion, slurred speech, seizures, and coma.

◆ Exercise. It turns out that exercise is not just good for your heart and lungs. It also does wonders for helping to process glucose. Again, your pancreas used to monitor the amount of glucose you would need to exercise, but now you will have to step in and take over that function. Before and after you exercise vigorously, you may need to check your blood glucose level and adjust your insulin accordingly.

◆ Be on the lookout for complications. In essence, diabetes is a glucose disorder. And because glucose is needed by just about every cell in your body, complications can develop. People with diabetes are vulnerable to problems with their circulatory system, nerve endings, kidneys, and eyes (see pages 143–154 for more information). Good glucose control will dramatically reduce the likelihood of complications.

Glucose meters
your diagnostic tools

One of the main jobs of the pancreas is to sense the presence of glucose in the blood. You will now need to take over that sensing job yourself. To do that, you will need to monitor the level of glucose in your blood at various times of the day. How do you do that? With a glucose meter, a device about the size of a pack of cards or a cell phone that tells you how much glucose is in your blood. To use the meter, you first insert a testing strip into it. The meter usually has a small liquid crystal display on the front like the one you see on a calculator. You use a small device called a lancet, which is about the size of a pen, to give your finger or forearm a small poke and draw a tiny drop of blood. Within 5 to 30 seconds you get a reading of your glucose level. Glucose-meter readings give you a good idea of whether your diabetes is under control at that particular moment.

You will want to keep your meter with you always and check your blood frequently. You typically test in the morning on an empty stomach (this is called a fasting test), before meals, an hour or two after meals, and before bed. The idea is to test frequently, rather than just when you think your blood sugar is high or low. For instance, some people with type 2 diabetes, whose blood sugar varies little, test just in the morning. Others, whose sugar rises and falls more dramatically, need to test more often, usually three to six times a day. Your doctor will let you know how often to test.

Your doctor will ask you to log your results in a small booklet and bring them to your next appointment. This will provide the best idea of what's going on with your diabetes and will allow your physician to make adjustments to your medicines (pills and/or insulin) with more confidence. If you can, try to keep tabs on your weight and feelings, too. (See pages 22–23 on creating a health journal.)

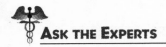

I have just been diagnosed with diabetes and am starting my treatment. Every time I have to prick my finger in public, I inevitably get some comment from someone. What can I do?

Doing daily finger sticks can be painful on many levels. It can irritate your finger, and it also interrupts your day—to say nothing of reminding you and others that you have a chronic illness that requires constant management. To avoid the prying eyes of others, you might try to find a private space to do your testing. Most people with diabetes test themselves in a bathroom.

However, you might also decide to take a completely different tack and be open about your illness, which can help normalize others' reaction to it. Some diabetes educators are trying to empower people to "come out of the closet" with their diabetes and do their testing in public as if it were an everyday act like tying a shoelace. Most onlookers are just curious and want to see how the monitor works. Often, they have a family member with diabetes and are interested in the new devices for self-care. The bottom line? You should do what makes you feel the most comfortable.

My doctor also wants me to have a test that gauges my blood sugar over the long term. What is that?

The most frequently used test is called Hemoglobin A_{1c}, which gives you an estimation of your average blood sugar over 60 to 90 days. Your doctor will request that you have blood drawn for a hemoglobin test every three months, regardless of whether you have type 1 or 2 diabetes. This test should give your doctor a general idea of how you are doing. Keep in mind that people with a lot of daily glucose highs and lows can also have a Hemoglobin A_{1c} result that appears normal.

All about insulin
there are several different types

Type 1 diabetes is essentially a disease in which the pancreas does not create enough insulin to help the body use sugar for energy. (Type 2 diabetes is mainly a disease of insulin resistance.) As your diabetes educator will tell you, the treatment for type 1 diabetes is elegantly simple: provide synthetic insulin to do the job the pancreas can no longer perform. Until recently, most diabetics used beef or pork insulin (or a mix) extracted from the pancreases of cows and pigs. Beef and pork insulin have saved many lives since they were introduced in the 1920s. Most people used them with no problems. But beef and pork insulin are not identical to human insulin. In some cases, skin irritation or an allergic reaction occurred.

In the late 1970s, researchers created human insulin in a lab. It is made from bacteria normally found in humans. These bacteria, such as *E. coli*, are genetically modified to produce insulin that is identical to human insulin. This is done by adding the gene that produces human insulin to the genes in *E. coli* bacteria. Then, the bacteria cells produce it just like any other enzyme. This can be done in large quantities, making the process of culturing the cells and extracting and purifying the insulin very inexpensive.

Researchers have also developed several different types of insulin to deal with the various insulin needs of those with diabetes. Insulin types are typically distinguished by how fast they start lowering glucose (called **onset** by researchers), when they work the best (**peak**), and how long they stay in your system (**duration**). Insulin with a fast onset is good for covering the spike in blood sugar that comes from carbohydrates in meals. Slow-onset insulin mimics the body's process of providing you with a slow drip of insulin throughout the day.

Insulin comes in one form: injection. People with type 1 diabetes use injectable insulin to control blood sugar, and so do an increasing number of people with type 2 diabetes.

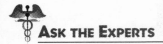

ASK THE EXPERTS

Why can't they make insulin in pill form?

The problem is that once insulin is ingested via a pill, it is destroyed by stomach enzymes. Researchers are working on ways to bypass this problem by creating inhalable insulin. See pages 54–55 for more on cutting-edge research.

Aren't the pills for type 2 diabetes insulin?

No. The pills used for type 2 diabetes are not synthetic insulin. Some work by stimulating the pancreas to produce more insulin, while others work by slowing the breakdown of starches. Still others work to curb the body's own production of sugar or increase the body's sensitivity to insulin. These pills are prescribed only for type 2 diabetes (see page 36 for more information).

Does it matter where I inject the insulin?

Where you inject insulin can affect the speed of absorption. An injection in your stomach is best because absorption there is the most constant. Your arm and leg muscles can also absorb insulin quickly, but this depends on how developed your muscles are. The bigger your muscles, the greater the rate of insulin absorption. You can also inject insulin into your buttocks. Bear in mind that you will need to alternate injection sites because injecting into the same place over and over eventually leads to slower absorption.

Insulin injections
today's syringes are nearly painless

Dealing with the fear of syringes is half the battle. Just know that today's syringes are remarkably fine and nearly painless. There was a time when insulin injections required boiling a glass syringe to sterilize it. And the needle was, in no one's estimation, thin or pain-free. Those days are, thankfully, long gone. Short needles are commonly used now to lessen pain from the injection.

Be careful when discarding used syringes. Place them in a plastic container, such as a large detergent bottle, that is not transparent. Tape it closed when full and discard it in your regular trash (not in the recycle bin).

The amount of insulin you draw is measured in "units." Here's how to inject insulin:

1. Some types of insulin, such as NPH (see page 33), appear cloudy. Vials of cloudy insulin should be rolled between your palms gently before use. Most clear insulins do not need to be rolled first.

2. Clean the top of the vial of insulin with an alcohol swab.

3. Before you draw any insulin, you first inject air (the same number of units as the insulin you will draw out) into the vial of insulin, which is about the size of a 35mm film cartridge.

4. Draw the insulin you'll be taking from the vial.

5. Use an alcohol swab to clean the area where you'll inject the insulin.

6. Pinch the skin to give yourself a little bit of fat into which you can inject. The point is to get the insulin into an area where it can be readily absorbed.

7. If sores later develop at any injection site, be sure to tell your doctor.

Common Types of Insulin

Which kind of insulin will you take? There are about 20 different types of insulin on the market today. Most insulin needs to be stored in the refrigerator. Here are the most common ones, along with some details on how they work. Note that the times—how long it takes for insulin to begin working, when it peaks, and the duration of its effect—are approximate, since they will vary from person to person.

Rapid-Acting Insulins

The fastest-acting insulins you can purchase are called lispro, sold under the brand name Humalog, and aspart, sold as Novolog. These types of insulin start working about 15 minutes after you take them. They are typically taken at mealtimes, to cover the carbs that you will eat. These insulins are also used in insulin pumps, for both the fast dose (bolus) and the continuous dose (basal). Aspart and lispro peak between 30 and 90 minutes after injection and can last up to five hours.

Short-Acting Insulins

Until recently, most people with diabetes who took insulin used a short-acting type called regular before meals and in insulin pumps. Regular insulin takes a bit longer to start working; it kicks in after about 30 minutes and peaks after two to four hours. Regular can last in your blood from four to eight hours.

Intermediate-Acting Insulins

Intermediate insulins, such as NPH and lente, act in 2 to 6 hours and peak between 4 and 14. They last in the blood for 14 to 20 hours.

Mixed Insulins

Some people mix rapid-acting and intermediate-acting insulins. You can purchase pre-mixed insulins so that you don't have to mix them yourself in the syringe by drawing insulin from two separate vials. You can buy insulin that contains, for example, 70 percent NPH and 30 percent Humalog. A 50-50 mix of the two insulins is also available.

Long-Acting Insulins

A relatively new insulin called glargine starts working 1 to 2 hours after injection, does not have a pronounced peak, and continues working for 24 hours. Many people have switched from NPH to glargine, which reduces incidences of low blood sugar while you are sleeping. Sold under the brand name Lantus, glargine is usually taken once or twice a day and acts as a background insulin, somewhat like the basal dose provided by an insulin pump. Lantus should not be mixed with any other type of insulin.

Less frequently used is ultralente insulin, which doesn't start working for 4 to 8 hours and stays in the blood 18 to 24 hours. It has a very small peak at 10 to 16 hours.

Your doctor will choose the right insulin for you. However, by knowing a bit about the insulins now available, you can discuss with your doctor how newer insulins can help you. For instance, most individuals used to take regular insulin before mealtime, and then wait 30 minutes for it to kick in before eating. But now lispro and aspart are much more common because they can be taken right before a meal.

Insulin pumps
they're expensive but can be so helpful

If you are not crazy about the idea of injections, or want more flexibility in terms of when you eat your meals, consider an insulin pump. About 25 percent of people with type 1 diabetes, and a small number of those with type 2, turn to insulin pumps to help control their blood sugar. An insulin pump provides a small, continuous dose of insulin, just like the pancreas does.

The pump is a battery-operated device, about the size of a pager, that is connected to a cartridge of insulin. The pump can be carried in your pocket or worn on your belt or under your clothing. Insulin pumps deliver two different doses of fast-acting insulin at different times.

◆ The basal dose is the small, continuous flow of insulin. You and your health-care professional determine the rate, when you first get your pump, by testing your blood sugar many times throughout the day.

◆ The bolus is a larger dose of mealtime insulin, which you control to cover the carbs you eat. A few minutes before you are ready to eat, you just press buttons on the pump to deliver the correct bolus dose.

There are a few downside factors to consider about pump therapy:

◆ With some pumps, you must insert a small, short needle into the tissue right under the skin of your abdomen every few days. This is the same place you would inject daily insulin; it's just that the pump needle stays there. (However, there are now some pumps that use thin plastic tubing and an "introducer" needle that is removed after insertion.)

◆ The pump must stay connected to you 24 hours a day.

◆ You need to keep an eye on the amount of insulin in the reservoir. You will want to make sure you have a syringe and backup insulin on hand in case your reservoir becomes empty unexpectedly.

- ◆ You need to watch the batteries. Pumps usually have an alarm that sounds if your batteries are getting low.

- ◆ Occasionally, people get a skin infection at the injection site.

- ◆ Pumps are more expensive than injections. The average price of a pump is $5,000, and supplies run about $1,500 a year. However, most insurers will cover the cost if you meet certain criteria.

If you don't really mind insulin injections, why use a pump? The reason is that insulin pumps offer the best glucose control of any therapy currently available for people who need daily insulin injections. The better the control, the lower the risk of complications. An insulin pump isn't for everyone, but many people who switch to the pump say they would never go back.

Getting used to being tethered to a pump can take time. The idea of having sex while you're connected to a pagerlike device doesn't seem terribly romantic. However, you can disconnect the pump at times like these or, for example, when you go swimming. That said, some pumps are now waterproof and can go in the shower; some can even be tucked away discreetly in your swimsuit.

FIRST PERSON INSIGHTS

Embracing the new

When my doctor suggested an insulin pump, it made me anxious. I didn't want people to know that I was always wearing this weird machine. My diabetes had always been easy to conceal, and I liked it that way. But my blood sugar was pretty out of control, so I grudgingly gave it a try. My first night with the pump, I slept more soundly than usual. In the morning, I felt better than I had in years and had much more energy. The pump adjusted to my need for insulin much better than injections ever did. I ate breakfast without giving myself a shot for the first time in five years. I sat in the kitchen and let that feeling sink in—no more shots, ever again!

—Sara S., New Haven, CT

Pills for type 2 diabetes
talk to your doctor about potential side effects

Diet and exercise can have a major impact on keeping your blood sugar in control. But, if you're like most people, you may need some medicinal help. People with type 2 diabetes often take one or more of a number of oral medications to help their bodies produce more insulin or use it more effectively. Here are some of the different drugs that can help:

◆ **Sulfonylureas** have been in use for more than 50 years. They stimulate the pancreas to produce more insulin.

◆ **Biguanides** reduce the amount of glucose released by the liver, and that helps keep your blood sugar lower. Metformin is a commonly prescribed biguanide.

◆ **Alpha-glucosidase inhibitors** help slow or halt the breakdown of starches and sugars. Acarbose is one of these.

◆ **Thiazolidinediones** help reduce insulin resistance. Rosiglitazone and Pioglitazone are common thiazolidinediones.

◆ **Meglitinides** stimulate your pancreas to make more insulin but are not the same as sulfonylureas. Nateglinide and Repaglinide are commonly prescribed meglitinides.

If you have type 1 diabetes, talk about oral medications probably sounds pretty good, especially compared to injections. The problem is that insulin cannot be taken orally because it would break down when it meets the acid in your stomach. Oral medications, for now, are primarily for individuals with type 2 diabetes.

Oral Hypoglycemics

Unfortunately, over time, oral diabetes medications begin to lose their effectiveness. It's not clear why, but it likely has to do with the pancreas becoming less effective as you age. Some people will need to take a combination of different drugs, or incorporate insulin injections in addition to pills, to control their blood sugar.

Some of these medications are taken just once or twice a day; others are taken at, or just before, meals. Talk to your doctor about when to take your diabetes pills.

	Generic Name	Brand Name	Potential Side Effects
Sulfonylureas	glipizide	Glucotrol or Glucotrol XL	Weight gain, mild stomach upset, alcohol intolerance, skin irritation, hypoglycemia
	glimepiride	Amaryl	
	tolbutamide	Orinase	
	tolazamide	Tolinase	
	acetohexamide	Dymelor	
	clorpropamide	Glucamide or Diabinese	
	glyburide	Diabeta, Glynase, and Micronase	
Alpha-glucosidase inhibitors	acarbose	Precose	Gas, bloating, diarrhea
	meglitol	Glyset	
Biguanides	metformin	Glucophage or Glucophage XR	Nausea, mild stomach upset, diarrhea, loss of appetite. People with kidney disease, liver disease, or heart failure and alcoholics should not take metformin. You might need to stop taking metformin for several days if you need an X-ray that involves dye.
Thiazolidinediones	rosiglitazone	Avandia	Weight gain, muscle fatigue, edema
	pioglitazone	Actose	
Meglitinides	repaglinide	Prandin	Weight gain and hypoglycemia
	nateglinide	Starlix	

Big benefits from exercise
exercise helps control blood sugar

You have a lot to do and think about when you have diabetes, and it's understandable that being told to add exercise to your new health regimen can seem like just another chore. If you are not already exercising regularly, a workout routine can be tough to start and tougher to continue. But a little physical activity can make a big difference and the benefits are dramatic, both in your day-to-day life and in the long term. Exercise keeps your blood sugar in check and helps keep your weight under control. Weight loss improves insulin resistance and can help reduce blood pressure. Getting some aerobic activity can also reduce the risk of heart disease and stroke. No small matter, this, since people with diabetes are at higher risk for heart disease, and elevated blood pressure increases the risk of kidney disease.

You don't need to run a marathon. Most experts agree that 30 minutes of heart-rate–elevating exercise every day is sufficient. A short walk each morning (or, ideally, twice a day) will work wonders. If you have other health problems that limit what you can do, talk to your diabetes educator; you might need something that benefits multiple conditions. Water aerobics, for example, is great exercise and can help alleviate the pain of arthritis and keep your glucose in check.

It can be very hard to get the ball rolling. For a lot of people, regular exercise is more daunting than insulin therapy. What you need to do is find an exercise routine you'll stick with. The trick is to find something you enjoy that doesn't feel like work. Meanwhile, start walking to do errands instead of driving, park farther away from the entrance if you drive, and take the stairs instead of the escalator.

Exercise and Blood Sugar

When you have diabetes, exercise can be both a pro and a con. You want to make sure your blood sugar does not drop too low while you exercise. If you need to eat continually to make up for lower blood sugar when you exercise, you can end up gaining weight. And, in some cases, exercising can actually make your blood sugar rise. Here are some strategies to help balance blood sugar and exercise:

◆ Check your blood sugar an hour before exercising.

◆ If your blood sugar is low, eat a small snack with a lot of carbohydrates to raise your blood sugar and protein to keep your blood sugar in the normal range. Half of a turkey sandwich or crackers with peanut butter (but watch the fat), may do the trick.

◆ If you take insulin, you can also reduce your rapid-acting dose to compensate for exercise.

◆ You will typically burn more calories on an empty stomach. But this will not work if your blood sugar is low. You might counter that by exercising after eating.

◆ Exercise can make the liver produce more glucose, which will raise your blood sugar level. So if your blood sugar is high (for example, over 250 mg/dl), it can go up when you exercise. In this case, it's best to delay exercising until your blood sugar level is normal.

Keep in mind that exercise can continue to lower your blood sugar well after you stop (for up to 12 hours, and in some cases 24). Check your blood sugar before bedtime and, if necessary, eat something with carbohydrates and protein in it to keep your blood sugar up. If you are not sure what to eat before bedtime, ask your diabetes educator to recommend something that you will enjoy.

Diet and weight loss
eat what you want, but watch the calories and carbs

Diet plays such an important role in dealing with diabetes that you will soon become an expert at proper nutrition. (For further information on food and diabetes, see pages 83–104.) No doubt you probably have some questions about diet and diabetes that you want answered right away. Here are some of the most frequently asked questions.

I can't even stay on a regular diet, so how am I supposed to deal with a restrictive diabetic diet?

There is actually no such thing as a diabetic diet. You don't have to eat only grapefruit for breakfast, or only a roll at lunch, like your coworker who is shedding pounds at a furious rate (but will gain them all back as soon as he or she goes off the diet). Keep an eye on the foods you love, but be sure to lower your consumption of carbohydrates. Your best way to lose a pound of fat is to reduce your caloric intake by about 500 calories a day, through a mix of diet and exercise. But it's most important that you watch your blood sugar levels and work to keep them in the normal range. If you take insulin, you must make sure to take enough to cover the carbohydrates.

Can I lower my blood sugar with diet alone?

Blood sugar levels in both type 1 and type 2 diabetes can be lowered by avoiding foods that are high in carbohydrates. That doesn't mean you will solve your insulin problem, however. Eating a diet low in sugar will help keep your blood sugar level low, and that's a good thing.

Are low-carbohydrate diets a fast way to lose weight?

With all this talk about the benefits of weight loss and watching your carbohydrate intake, you might be tempted to try a diet that helps you drop weight quickly by cutting out carbohydrates. These high-protein, low-carbohydrate diets can lead to pretty dramatic weight loss, as well as an overall reduction in blood sugar levels, which makes such diets appealing. However, all that extra protein can make the kidneys work harder than usual. Since people with diabetes are at a higher risk of developing kidney disease, this is a concern. So stay away from fad diets. You want a slow and steady weight loss of, say, three to four pounds a month. Besides, a balanced diet is easier to maintain. Whatever you do, it's extremely important that you discuss any dietary change with your doctor, diabetes educator, or dietitian before making major adjustments.

Do I have to give up alcohol?

In a word, no. But you do need to watch your intake: not only how much you drink but when. Most alcohol is made of fermented fruit or grain—both of which contain carbohydrates. It's the grape juice in wine and the fermented barley in beer that can elevate blood sugar levels. If you are taking insulin or oral medications for diabetes, you should drink only at meals and never on an empty stomach. The rule is no more than two drinks a day for men, one drink a day for women. For more information on diabetes and alcohol, see pages 98–99.

Can I eat sugar—as in table sugar or a doughnut?

In the past, if you had diabetes, you were told to swear off sugar, unless the amount of sugar in your blood dropped too low and you needed to bring it up quickly. These days, most experts agree that your diet can include simple sugar, such as that found in candy or cakes, in moderation. Moderation is important because foods high in sugar are also high in calories. If you decide to eat sweets, the trick is to make them part of your meal plan. Here's what the American Diabetes Association says: "Don't pass up a slice of birthday cake. Instead, at the next meal, eat a little less bread or potato and be sure to take a brisk walk to burn some calories."

Smart treatment tips
keep your medications and glucose tabs handy

Problems with blood sugar levels can arise at any time, and you need to be prepared for them. When your blood sugar is low, you need about 15 grams of fast-acting carbohydrates. Glucose tablets are inexpensive, fast-acting doses of sugar that taste like fruit-flavored candy. If food is not readily available, these tablets will do the trick.

It's a good idea to keep a container of glucose tabs in your purse, in the car, at your desk, on the night table—anywhere you might be caught off guard with a low-blood-sugar episode. Glucose tabs are particularly handy because they're lower in calories than, say, a can of soda. And, because they are not as tasty as a chocolate bar, they are also less likely to be noshed by your friends, kids, or sweets-loving spouse. On the off chance that you feel too faint to eat a glucose tab, you should have a syringe of glucagon at hand. Once injected, it will immediately raise your blood sugar. You will need to tell family members how to inject it in the case of an emergency. (Some people with diabetes keep a tub of cake frosting on hand; the frosting can be smeared on their gums if they are unable to eat.)

Next, you need to keep your medication, meters, glucose tabs, and a glucagon emergency kit on you at all times. Yes, that can be awkward when you want to go out footloose and fancy-free, but you never know when you might get stranded and need insulin. It's especially important to keep these items with you when traveling.

And you need to tell friends and coworkers about your illness in case you run into trouble and need medical help. Be straightforward. (See pages 164–165 for how to talk about your diabetes.) If your child has diabetes, make sure to let the teacher know that your child may act in unusual ways when blood sugar levels are high or low, and explain how to help your child overcome them—for instance, by chewing a glucose tablet.

ID Bracelets for Diabetics

As if having diabetes isn't tough enough, you will occasionally be reminded by your doctor or diabetes educator that things can get worse. Worse, as in you are in a serious accident and cannot tell the people who are trying to help you that you have diabetes. Or you lose consciousness from very low blood sugar or very high blood sugar and dehydration. How do you let helpful strangers know that you have diabetes, and not some other affliction? The solution is to wear some sort of ID. MedicAlert, a nonprofit organization, sells bracelets and pendants that provide information about your condition when you cannot. The bracelet lets an emergency responder know that you have diabetes and provides a toll-free phone number to call. When contacted, MedicAlert sends the emergency team your medical history.

MedicAlert is relatively inexpensive, starting at $35 for a year of the service, which includes a stainless-steel bracelet or pendant (though you can spend as much as $650 for a fancy gold designer one!). Contact MedicAlert at 888-633-4298 or go to **www.medicalert.org**.

FIRST PERSON INSIGHTS

The cold, hard truth

It was a crisp winter morning and looked like a great day for a hike. I packed a few supplies and set out. By noon, a snowstorm had started up. I knew I had to turn back, but by the time I got to a road, I could barely see. I walked for miles and felt the cold seeping in. I had eaten all my snacks and was shaking badly. I found a bus shelter, but the city was deserted. Finally, a cop drove by. He must have known I was in deep trouble because he immediately took me to the hospital. By that time, I was out of it. I told them I had diabetes and they gave me a glucose shot. The doctor said I was lucky. I had no idea that hours out in the cold could cause such problems. It finally dawned on me that my diabetes is a serious condition and that I need to have a backup plan at all times.

—Tim R., Fargo, ND

Helpful resources

*The I Hate to Exercise Book for
People with Diabetes*
by Charlotte Hayes

**Emergency Identification
MedicAlert
www.medicalert.org**

**Children with Diabetes
www.childrenwithdiabetes.com**

CHAPTER 3

Using the Internet

Top health sites for laypeople
the best sites to start with

You have had the tests. And you have been given a diagnosis and perhaps even begun your treatment. If you are like most people, your first instinct is to find out everything there is to know about diabetes. This is a useful instinct—hold on to it. You don't need to become a diabetes expert; your goal is to become an informed, active patient. But first, a word of advice: Don't just turn on your computer and start by typing "diabetes" into the main search engines. The information you will get can and will overwhelm you. Instead, turn to the sites listed below to ground you in the basics about diabetes. If you don't have Internet access at home, many public libraries have Internet-access stations that you can use for half an hour or more at a stretch. Here are three good starting points:

HealthScout
www.healthscout.com
The HealthScout Network provides health-encyclopedia information and focused news reports for big Web sites like Yahoo, USA Today, and NBCi. You can see at a glance that it's supported by advertising, but that doesn't get in the way of the content.

Your first port of call should be HealthScout's encyclopedia. The quickest way to get to the right place is to enter a keyword or two in the search box on the HealthScout's home page. What you will get is a listing of articles and their dates, as well as a percentage figure at the end that tells you how relevant the article is to your keyword. If it's 100 percent, the article is definitely worth a look.

EndocrineWeb

www.endocrineweb.com

You can tell by the name that EndocrineWeb is going to get a little more technical. Your body's endocrine system includes all your glands, and EndocrineWeb covers them all. Enter "diabetes" in the search field and you will be ready for your course on your disease. EndocrineWeb's pages are nicely illustrated. It reads like an intelligent magazine article rather than a crusty academic tome. The articles are just long enough and just technical enough to help you "get" the whole thing.

FIRST PERSON INSIGHTS

In the know

My wife signed up for a diabetes e-mail list, where each message went to everyone who had signed up for the list. After a few weeks, she began to bring home tips that were new to me. She helped me find a new glucose meter that required just a tiny drop of blood and was painless to use. She read about a new type of insulin that sounded like it might help me avoid low blood sugar in the night. I introduced the idea to my doctor, who enthusiastically prescribed the insulin to me. My wife was concerned that some of the people on the list were feeling really down and had problems that were far worse than mine. She thought I might find the list discouraging. But when we moved and my wife no longer had her office e-mail account, I signed up for the group. I didn't find it scary at all, and I enjoyed offering support and the tips I had learned to new people on the list. (For more about diabetes e-mail lists, see pages 64–65.)

—Roger M., Richmond, VA

Top medical-research sites
go to these for clinical information

Once you've got a basic grounding in your diabetes, you will be ready for something more substantial. Again, avoid doing a general search and go instead to the established medical sites. There are two basic types of sites: those that are maintained by a specific medical school or clinic, and the big medical search engines that are supported by the U.S. government.

Medical institutions

Universities and clinics often provide outreach sites for health issues, and academic resources are rigorously checked for accuracy. Here are some of the bigger medical sites run by institutions:

InteliHealth
www.intelihealth.com

Johns Hopkins University's excellent and easy-to-understand collection of journal databases also has a medical dictionary and expert Q&As.

Mayo Clinic
www.mayoclinic.com

The respected clinic's Web site does a great job of making health and medical issues easy to understand.

National Institutes of Health's Medline
www.nlm.nih.gov/medlineplus/

The prime source of clinical and patient-oriented information. Sometimes tough, but deep and useful.

National Institutes of Health's Healthfinder
www.healthfinder.gov/

Medical search engines

Search engines embedded in a reliable medical site are the quickest way to get good information from that site and sometimes from other sites that are affiliated with it. The pool you are searching is small, but because of that, you get the most relevant results. Some examples of medical search engines:

Healthfinder
www.healthfinder.gov/
A publication of the U.S. government's National Institutes of Health, Healthfinder's search engine finds pages from prescreened, authoritative sites. The content often doesn't go very deep, but it's written in an accessible way.

Medline
www.nlm.nih.gov/medlineplus/
Another site provided by the National Institutes of Health, Medline has a great deal of clinical information. Enter your search terms here, and you will get results with deep research from an encyclopedic government-run source.

Smart searching tips: Put quote marks around phrases (as in "blood sugar"), and most search engines will exclude results that include isolated uses of each of the words. Also, if you put a minus sign in front of words that tend to yield irrelevant results, the search engine will leave out all sites on that topic. For example, if you want to find sites about living with diabetes as an adult only, you should type in: "living with diabetes"-juvenile.

Nonprofit organizations
check out the advocacy groups

Nonprofit institutions and agencies dedicated to the study, cure, or relief of a particular ailment are another good source of reliable online information. They are not all patient-oriented, and they are sometimes contradictory (because professionals love to argue about details), but they can provide very helpful information. You can also use these sites to trade tips and chat online with other people with diabetes or even arrange to meet them in person. The Juvenile Diabetes Research Foundation, which focuses on type 1 diabetes, holds annual bike and walking fund-raisers for diabetes research. The American Diabetes Association holds get-out-the-message fund-raisers, as well as the Kiss-a-Pig event, where the big winner gets to, well, kiss a pig. Sounds silly, but it's held in 50 cities and raises millions of dollars a year.

American Diabetes Association
www.diabetes.org
The Diabetes.org Web site presents health, diet, and lifestyle information and recommendations for individuals with type 1 and type 2 diabetes in simple language. Very importantly, the organization acts as an advocate for people with diabetes in Washington, D.C. When you join the ADA, a subscription to its monthly magazine, *Diabetes Forecast*, is part of the bargain. The site could provide more features for direct communication among people with diabetes, but you'll find more of these community features on pages 64–65.

Juvenile Diabetes Research Foundation
www.jdrf.org
The Juvenile Diabetes Research Foundation, started more than 30 years ago by the parents of a child with diabetes, promotes type 1 diabetes advocacy and education. The JDRF is a great starting point for type 1 research. The organization and its efforts at fund-raising and education are top-

notch, though, like the ADA site, it could offer more community features, such as chats and bulletin boards.

Insulin-Free World Foundation
www.insulin-free.org

If you're interested in cutting-edge research, support, and advice from other individuals with diabetes, the Insulin Free Foundation is the place to go. The site incorporates online chats (where you can type instant messages to other people with diabetes at set meeting times) and lectures on islet and pancreas transplants. The down-to-earth approach of this site has improved the lives of many people with diabetes.

International Diabetes Federation
www.idf.org

The International Diabetes Federation offers a worldwide outlook on diabetes. The site focuses on the impact of diabetes around the world and provides information about trends, care, and prevention for people with diabetes in more than 200 countries.

Doctors and Internet-Savvy Patients

Some doctors become alarmed when patients come in with reams of printouts from the Internet. While it's true that some sites cannot be trusted, a number of medical Web sites have a formal panel of medical advisers—just like the physicians' favorite reading material, *The New England Journal of Medicine*. Your goal is to enter a dialogue with your doctor about your health. He will know you mean business if instead of saying something vague like "I read something on the Internet," you say "An article published on the American Diabetes Association's Web site says . . ."

Government agencies
going to the source

These agencies and their Web sites provide useful general information on diabetes as well as the latest scientific literature. If you need a quick rundown on, say, the latest diabetes pills, or you want a straight-talk approach to diet and exercise, you can usually find it here. Most of the information is written in a friendly tone.

National Institute of Diabetes and Digestive and Kidney Disease
www.niddk.nih.gov

The National Institutes of Health has conducted medical research for more than 100 years. The National Institute of Diabetes and Digestive and Kidney Disease, part of the NIH, hosts a Web site full of general information and research. You can find the latest on treatments, side effects, and physiology at this simple, well-organized site. Need a primer on the effects of high blood sugar on the kidneys? How about a quick definition of *starch* ("another name for a carbohydrate, one of the three main nutrients in food")? It's all here. Note that some of the information is presented in Adobe Acrobat's .pdf format. You can download Acrobat Reader for free at **www.adobe.com**. While you're at the NIH site, check out Medline, a comprehensive database of all sorts of medical information, including an illustrated medical encyclopedia: **www.nlm.nih.gov/medlineplus**.

Medfetch.com
www.medfetch.com

Medfetch alerts you to new medical information by e-mail. You type in what you're looking for and Medfetch e-mails you abstracts and citations from medical journals when it finds articles that match your search. You could, for instance, search for just "diabetes" to find new general information. Or you could run a multiword search, such as "islet and transplant." Note that this is heavy reading.

Food and Drug Administration
www.fda.gov
www.fda.gov/diabetes

Since the FDA regulates foods and medical products you use to treat diabetes, you can find some pretty interesting new products on the site as they are approved. A recent survey of the site showed an approval notice of a children's watch that measures blood sugar levels over the day and a new over-the-counter home testing kit for glycated hemoglobin (which measures blood sugar over three to four months). The site also provides the text of medical-research reports.

Researching Complementary Therapies

The Internet is also an excellent resource when you would like to find out about complementary therapies (for more on complementary therapies, see pages 105–118). For instance, go to **www.askJeeves.com** and type in "diabetes" and the name of the therapy you are interested in. You will be taken to related Web pages. Another approach is to check out some tried-and-true complementary-therapy sites. Here are a few:

1. Dr. Weil online. Dr. Andrew Weil is an AMA-trained doctor who has been one of the leading forces behind the holistic-medicine movement. His site, **drweil.com**, covers all sorts of disorders and offers advice on various types of alternative treatments. When you click on his site and type in your particular disorder, you may find that the good doctor has some alternative-therapy advice that may help.

2. Another useful site is the Healthplus Web page. This site is composed of a consortium of alternative therapies. Click on it to learn about all the various therapies available, whether yoga or light therapy. It also has a tab for finding practitioners. Go to **www.healthplusweb.com**.

3. Another site, **www.Healthy.net**, has a referral service that will point you to doctors who practice "integrative medicine," meaning they combine traditional AMA medicine with alternative treatments.

On top of the news
staying in the know

Innovations in diabetes care really picked up speed in the mid-1990s. Since then, we've seen the first synthetic human insulins, less painful blood-testing meters, more effective diabetes pills, and promising steps toward a cure. The next 10 years look to be even more exciting, as researchers develop new treatments for type 1 and type 2 diabetes. But how to keep up? There's no shortage of diabetes news on the Web. Here are a few places that do a particularly good job of keeping you in the know:

Diabetes Portal
www.diabetesdailynews.org

The Diabetes Portal combines content from several informative sites in one place. You'll find bulletin boards, chats, and lots of news and communication between the sites and readers. The site is smartly and enthusiastically managed by people who have diabetes and those who care about them. The Diabetes Daily News area links to current articles about diabetes from wire services. The site also features a "news feed"—links to stories about diabetes treatment and research from other news sources on the Web.

Children with Diabetes
www.childrenwithdiabetes.com

The Children with Diabetes site frequently updates its news page with links to research reports and articles on treatment for young people with diabetes, as well as personal stories of children dealing with diabetes from newspapers and magazines around the country. You can access the news page from the Children with Diabetes home page.

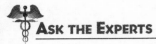

ASK THE EXPERTS

I sometimes read about new treatments, and then they seem to vanish. What's up?

The media tend to jump on the latest new treatments, often suggesting a cure is imminent. In the 1970s a popular science magazine ran the headline "Just Around the Corner" on its cover, in reference to a cure for diabetes through islet-cell transplants. We're still waiting. Articles that herald breakthroughs in diabetes should be read with a skeptical eye. It takes about 10 years for any new treatment to undergo the appropriate testing before the FDA will approve it.

I'm shopping for a new glucose meter. Where can I find independent reviews?

The Children with Diabetes site does a nice job of reviewing glucose-testing meters. *Diabetes Forecast*, the magazine of the ADA, also does a good annual review of meters. Outside the United States, glucose meters report results in mmol/L (millimoles per liter) rather than mg/dl (milligrams per deciliter). You can find a conversion chart here: **www.joslin.harvard.edu/education/ library/ConversionTable.shtml**.

I've read some scary information about certain diabetes pills. Where can I get more information?

You can read about the latest diabetes pills available at the Web site for the National Institute of Diabetes and Digestive and Kidney Diseases (NIDDK), which is part of the NIH: **www.niddk.nih.gov/health/ diabetes/pubs/med/specific.htm**.

Diet and exercise
eating smart

Hit the Web and you can find recipes for healthy meals that are quick to prepare and learn how various foods affect your blood sugar. These Web sites can also help teach you how to live healthier, keep blood sugar levels in control, and lose weight.

Glycemic Index
www.diabetes.about.com/library/mendosag:/nmedosag.html
The glycemic index (GI) determines how quickly carbohydrates are converted to glucose. Lower-GI foods produce less of a spike in your blood sugar. Some complex carbohydrates, such as a baked potato, raise your blood sugar faster than table sugar does. You can make subtle food substitutions that can help keep blood sugar in the normal range—for instance, replacing white rice and white bread with basmati rice and whole-grain breads. Rick Mendosa, a writer who specializes in diabetes, provides an excellent introduction to the glycemic index, as well as a list of foods and their GI values.

FDA Nutrient Database
www.nal.usda.gov/fnic/foodcomp
Want to know how much protein there is in an egg white? how many carbs in a granola bar? You can search for the nutritional content of any food by using the FDA's nutrient database.

Diabetic Gourmet
www.diabeticgourmet.com/recipes
You're home from work, hungry, and in need of a quick and tasty meal. Hop on your computer and find a recipe fast. This site's recipe archive breaks down the nutritional values of each meal and includes prep time. You can search by category, such as appetizers and vegetarian, regional, or ethnic cuisine. You can also sign up for an e-mail newsletter that will deliver a recipe to your inbox each day.

Up and running

You can find sites on the Web that will help you develop exercise goals and programs that may make you feel better and improve the effectiveness of your insulin. Here are some sites to help you shed stress, lower your blood pressure, and speed up your metabolism.

Diabetes Exercise and Sports Association
www.diabetes-exercise.org

This nonprofit organization (also called DESA) can put you in touch with diabetes and exercise support groups, and you can trade information through its online message boards. DESA promotes local bike tours and offers tips from individuals with diabetes who successfully handle diet and exercise.

The American Diabetes Association's Exercise Guide
www.diabetes.org/exercise

The ADA presents simple, authoritative advice for getting started, nutrition information, frequently asked questions, and safety tips (for example, you should have a medical exam before you start an exercise program and check your blood sugar during exercise). A recent update to the site provides a link to an audio program on diabetes and exercise, which you can listen to over your Internet connection.

About.com Diabetes Exercise
http://results.about.com/diabetes

The diabetes area of the About.com site features links to sites that cover diabetes and exercise from around the Web. You'll find a wide range of information, including tips for children with diabetes.

Keeping useful records
create your own research portfolio

It's easy to get lost when you first go online to learn about your new condition. There are all sorts of sites out there. One way to make sense of it all is to keep notes on where you travel on the Internet highway. In fact, you can use your computer to chart your journey. Here's how:

Bookmark important pages. Great, you just hit the motherlode of information—a page with tons of handy links and lots of good, solid information. Instead of stopping to write down the name of the site, save time and bookmark it! Every Web browser has the ability to let you save the location of favorite Web pages. All you have to do is go to the Web site you want to note, go up to the toolbar, and click on the tab that will save the site in the Bookmarks pull-down menu. In Internet Explorer, click on Favorites; in America Online, click on Favorite Places; and in Netscape, click on Bookmarks. To access that favorite Web page, all you need to do is look through your list of favorite sites or bookmarks and click on it.

Print out important bits of information. When you find a page with a lot of relevant information on it, print it out and file it in your health journal (see page 22). Use a three-hole punch to organize your printouts tidily in a three-ring binder. As your binder fills up, categorize your printouts by topic: medicine, specialists, alternative therapies, and so on. This will make it easier to find the information.

Save your ink!

You don't have to print out a whole Web page—you can drag your computer mouse across just the bit that interests you, and then print out only your selection: Click on File, then Print; in the Print box, click next to the word Selection. Then click on the OK button and you'll have a nice short printout.

Evaluating Web Sites

Not all the information on the Web is accurate. Before you start building up your health journal, make sure the Web pages you want to add are providing reliable information. Some sites may contain outdated facts, misinformation, poor research, urban legends, propaganda, and outright lies. How can you tell what's good and what's not? Use this checklist.

1. Check the date. In a book or newspaper, you can always check the publication date to find out whether the information is current. On the Web, not every page has the publication date. The better medical sites do. If you don't see a date, don't trust any figures the page calls "current."

2. Check out the source. Most articles online have bylines with the writer's name. If you haven't heard of the writer or don't know his or her reputation, feed the name into a search engine (see page 49) and see what else carries the byline. Also, a good medical paper always backs up its statements with sources and bibliographies. Check any article for sources and links to other sites.

3. Check out the publisher. Look at the Web address of any article you are evaluating. Is it a name you recognize—a well-known clinic, foundation, or government site? If not, look around for a link labeled "About this site," or something like that, and see who is behind it all.

4. Don't be put off by advertising. Advertising is a fact of life on the Web. One exception: If a site seems to be selling something in its articles, move on. You can't trust advertorials on television, so don't trust your health to them online either.

Better searching
start your engines

Now that you are up to speed on diabetes, you can do some general searching if you want. Check out Google (**www.google.com**), which gets high marks for effective searching and is used about 70 million times a day. Some other search engines include AltaVista (**www.altavista.com**), All The Web (**www.alltheweb.com**), and Lycos (**www.lycos.com**) which lets you enter searches in the form of a simple question.

An alternative approach is to use a directory. A directory uses human intelligence to select sites that are deemed useful, rather than simply listing every site available. A well-known directory is LookSmart (**www.look smart.com**). The diabetes area of About.com (see page 57) is another good directory, scrutinized by a moderator who follows the subject closely.

Need a new doctor? The Web site of the American Association of Clinical Endocrinologists offers an online physician finder at **www.aace.com/ memsearch.php**. The American Medical Association also maintains a database which you can search for an endocrinologist, at **www.ama-assn.org**. The Diabetes Physician Recognition Program (**www.ncqa.org/dprp**) only lists doctors who meet strict guidelines for care and patient satisfaction.

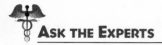

How can I tell if the information I'm reading is from a reliable source?

Look for the original source of information. Web sites that spout figures without linking directly to the original source are suspect.

I see a lot of diabetes-related stuff for sale. Are these things effective?

As you surf the Internet, you will come across plenty of online ads for "miracle" herbal medicines, supplements, and even "cures" for diabetes. But consider the source. It's depressing, but these sites are most often just trying to make a fast buck from an eager audience.

I seem to get a lot of irrelevant results when I search. Where do I find the really helpful material?

The first step in making your searches more successful is to use a good search engine, like those mentioned in this chapter. Once you find a search engine you like, try these tips:

◆ It's important to use precise search terms or keywords. The more words you type in, the more specific your search will be. Entering more keywords increases the relevancy of what you get in return but also limits the number of results you will get. Try a broad search first, then narrow down the results by adding search terms.

◆ Each search engine typically has a link that takes you to an "advanced" search form. There you can enter words you do *not* want to see. For example, you could refine your search by excluding the words "type 1" if you only want to see information on type 2 diabetes.

◆ Put quotes around common phrases. Searching for "glucose monitors" will yield pages that refer specifically to this testing device, rather than pages on glucose in general.

Online support
welcome to the world of newsgroups

To many people, newsgroups are just as important as Web sites when it comes to the Internet. They are lively, online communities of people with mutual interests in every subject under the sun, and their e-mails are stored online for you to browse. Newsgroups are a place to ask questions, pick up advice, and post your own so that others can benefit. On the opposite page, you'll see how to view newsgroups, step by step.

Once you are logged on to a newsgroup, you can post your own message by e-mailing it to the newsgroup, then check back in a day or so and probably find several helpful responses. Here are a few newsgroups you might like to check out:

alt.support.diabetes
alt.support.diabetes.kids
alt.food.diabetic

As you scan the groups, you may notice that some responses to questions contain derisive comments. Don't let Internet know-it-alls get you down. Take time to read the Frequently Asked Questions (also known as "FAQs"), available for most newsgroups, so that you don't ask a question that's been answered many times before. The FAQ for misc.health.diabetes can be found at **www.faqs.org/faqs/diabetes/**.

If you don't feel like dealing with a newsgroup, you can also look for online bulletin boards at Web sites, which work pretty much the same way. You post a question, others answer. Or you can just read up on what's been posted before. Several of the Web sites at **www.diabetesportal.com**, mentioned earlier in this chapter, offer helpful bulletin boards where people with diabetes can talk shop and socialize.

Newsgroup management

Ready to see if newsgroups are for you? All you need is an Internet connection and a Web browser, such as Internet Explorer, which is bundled free with every PC. It's also the browser used by AOL. Open your Web browser and try Google Groups. Go to the site **http://groups.google.com**

If you're not sure where to begin, you can type in words that describe what you want to know. Google finds specific messages that contain those words and points you to one or more newsgroups that use the words you entered. You can choose to view all the messages in the newsgroup, or just read a specific message that matches your search.

Let's say you want to find out about less painful glucose-testing meters. In the Google Groups search box, type "painless glucose testing." Now click the Google Search button. The results appear in your Web browser. Click the subject line of a message to view it.

What if you want to post your own message or a follow-up message to one you have read? To post using Google, you first need to sign up for a free account. Once you fill in the registration form, there are two ways to post a new message:

1. Click the Post a New Message link from the main newsgroup page, or

2. When viewing someone else's message, click Post a Follow-up to This Message.

Type your message and click the Preview Message button to see what it looks like. Or click Post Message to send it on its way.

Mailing lists
you've got friends

No one could blame you for feeling down or confused about the hassle of dealing with diabetes. Mailing lists are a good way to find out how others are faring in similar situations. A typical message arrives in your inbox from someone who is having trouble and is frustrated. Very quickly the group responds, sending e-mails with advice, tips, and encouragement to everyone on the list. You benefit from the public exchange of information, and you can join in with your thoughts just by sending an e-mail to the list.

DM-Life (Life with Diabetes Mellitus)

This is an engaging list composed of diabetes individuals who are almost unfailingly sympathetic and helpful to others. Curious about why your blood sugar jumps after drinking a cup of coffee? Not sure about switching to a new type of insulin? Having trouble with an infection that won't heal? Drop an e-mail, quick, and you will get smart advice and tips. To subscribe, send an e-mail to **dmlife-subscribe@yahoo.com**.

The Diabetes List

Typical messages discuss how people vary in their blood sugar reactions to certain foods, insulin preferences, and attitudes toward individuals with diabetes. Traffic is heavy, with messages arriving throughout the day. If that's too hectic for you, try the digest version, which collects the messages into one e-mail sent out just once a day. Instructions are on the opposite page.

Children with Diabetes mailing lists
www.childrenwithdiabetes.com/people/mailinglists.htm
The excellent Children with Diabetes site offers a handful of mailing lists based on different interests. These include lists for younger children and teens, as well as for parents of children with diabetes. There is a list for people with diabetes who are watching their weight, health professionals, and lists for people in the U.K., New Zealand, and Australia. The site also offers

free, Web-based e-mail addresses you can use for your mailing lists, to keep them separate from your regular e-mail. You can sign up for the Children with Diabetes mailing list by going to the Web page shown here.

Mailing-list management

When you sign up for a diabetes mailing list, you might soon find it overwhelming. The sheer volume of messages sent daily can discourage you from keeping up with the list. You can set up mailing lists to deliver messages one at a time, or you might prefer to receive a single message containg all the collected e-mails, which is called a daily digest.

If you wanted to subscribe to the digest version of the Diabetes List's digest, you would first need to sign up for the regular e-mail digest. Then send an e-mail to **dmlife-digest@yahoogroups.com** with the following in the body of the message: subscribe diabetes digest. Other mailing lists have similar directions for subscribing to the digest version; try checking the Preferences or Options menu on the relevant Web sites.

Another way to control the flow of messages to your inbox is to sign up for one of the many free e-mail accounts available. You view and send mail through a Web site. The benefit is that it helps you keep your mailing list messages separate from your personal and business correspondence. The downside is that reading mail on a Web site can be slow compared to using your office e-mail account, for example, or America Online. Still, the price is right. You can sign up for free, Web-based e-mail accounts at Yahoo (**http://mail.yahoo.com**) or Hotmail (**www.hotmail.com**), or at the Children with Diabetes site (**www.cwdmail.com**).

Helpful resources

After Any Diagnosis
by Carol Svec

The Health Resource
www.theheathresources.com
Tel: 800-949-0090
You don't have to search the
Internet yourself. There are a number of companies that offer this
service for a fee. One such company,
called The Health Resource, will do
a custom extensive Internet
research complilation that is spe-
cialized to your diagnosis. Their
Internet specialists will then comb
through the Internet and other
sources and locate medical articles
or information geared toward your
specific situation, including main-
stream, experimental, and alternative treatments, along with top specialists. In a week to 10 days, you
will receive a hard copy of their
findings in a bound booklet, complete with glossary. Prices range
from $150 to $400.

CHAPTER 4

Putting Your Team Together

Your primary care doctor
do you need another?

Your primary care doctor (also known as your family doctor or general practitioner) is probably the one who diagnosed your diabetes in the first place. This doctor was the one who picked up on your symptoms, spoke those words that you will always remember, and calmed your early fears about your treatment. This is the doctor who knows you best and, ideally, is the one you want to help you care for your diabetes.

That's fine if your diabetes is well controlled. Your primary care doctor can likely treat it. The job is pretty straightforward. Your doctor will chart your progress, prescribe and make adjustments to your medicine, check for any signs of problems, and, if problems arise, refer you to a specialist. Your diabetes aside, you will still need your family doctor nearby if you come down with other, more common ailments, such as an ear or a sinus infection or the flu—not to mention for monitoring your blood pressure, cholesterol, and kidney function closely.

However, if diabetes is not your only health concern—if you also have heart disease, for instance—you may want to be referred to a diabetes specialist known as an endocrinologist. Chances are, you will still see your primary care doctor for checkups. Just be sure to keep your doctor in the loop about your diabetes treatment.

Tips for Choosing a Primary Care Physician

Finding a new doctor or switching doctors can be nerve-racking at the best of times, doubly so if you have diabetes. But it happens. If you locate to a new town, or take a new job with a different health insurer or HMO than your previous employer used, you can find yourself shopping for a new doctor to entrust with this crucial new factor in your life.

How to find a new doctor:

▲ Start with your former doctor; chances are, he or she will be able to refer you to someone.

▲ Call the local hospital to see if it has a diabetes educator or dietitian on staff (for more on this, see pages 72–73). These professionals work closely with diabetes specialists and can help you find one.

▲ Call your local hospital's referral line. They will refer you to doctors in the area who are taking on new patients.

Remember that under the Health Insurance Portability and Accountability Act, which took effect in April 2003, you have the right to a copy of your medical records. Before you switch doctors, get a copy and correct any errors. Make several duplicates to give to your new primary-care physician and other doctors you may be seeing. Be sure to add the corrected records to your health journal (see page 22).

Endocrinologist
a doctor who specializes in glands and hormones

An endocrinologist is a medical doctor who specializes in ailments of the endocrine system, a set of glands that make hormones. These various glands and their hormones control a number of key bodily functions. For instance, the thyroid gland releases hormones to regulate your energy level, and the adrenal cortex releases the stress hormones that allow you to respond to potentially threatening situations. In the case of diabetes, it's the pancreas and the hormone insulin that regulate your blood sugar.

The endocrine system is complex. To become an endocrinologist, a doctor has to complete four years of medical school, and then three or more years of training in internal medicine and two additional years of specialty training in endocrinology. After that, this doctor will have to pass the very demanding medical boards (or tests) in endocrinology in order to be board certified.

What should you look for in an endocrinologist? Keep in mind that a number of endocrinologists devote their practice to a specific gland; for instance, a thyroidologist specializes in diseases of the thyroid. Those who specialize exclusively in diabetes care are called **diabetologists.** A diabetologist will help you make the important decisions about your diabetes care. This doctor will see you at least twice a year (or every few months if you take insulin) and work with you to prevent diabetic complications.

Your endocrinologist should be someone who puts you at ease. You need to be able to speak frankly about your lifestyle, home and work habits, and likes and dislikes. You need to be comfortable informing your doctor about how your treatment is going. If you have to contact your doctor about your treatment outside of scheduled appointments, the doctor or staff should respond within a reasonable amount of time.

Finding an Endocrinologist

Because your endocrinologist is going to be a Very Important Person in your life for many years to come, it's wise to take time now to make sure that he or she is Dr. Right.

When you go to your first appointment, there are a few questions you can ask to help determine whether you and this endocrinologist will work well together. Here are some to start with:

◆ Do you specialize in diabetes care?

◆ What percentage of your patients have diabetes?

◆ Do you see primarily people with type 1 or type 2 diabetes?

◆ How often do you like to see your diabetes patients? Every three months? More often?

◆ What happens in an emergency when you are not available?

There are no correct answers to these questions, but it's important that you get the answers you need and want. And if you are having trouble managing your blood sugar, you will want to find an experienced endocrinologist who works with diabetes patients daily.

Diabetes educator
knowledge is power

A certified diabetes educator is a nurse, dietitian, pharmacist, or, in some cases, physical therapist or social worker who has received intensive training and passed a rigorous written test in order to work with people with diabetes. The educator is there to make your life easier, working in tandem with your doctor (whether your primary physician or endocrinologist) to help you monitor your care, solve problems, and find a treatment plan (exercise, diet, and medicine) that works for you, rather than imposing hard-and-fast rules that you cannot handle. It's likely that you were introduced to an educator when you were first diagnosed.

Some educators are dietitians. More often, however, the educator works with a dietitian, perhaps in the same office. You might meet both at the same time, and you might not think to see one again. Here's what an educator can offer you:

◆ An educator can give you more time to discuss problems with your treatment plan and find solutions that fit your lifestyle. Rarely is the educator as rushed as your doctor. You can make a quick phone call to an educator with a question, or you can go to the office, often at a nearby hospital, to discuss how you are doing and review adjustments to diet, exercise, and medicine.

◆ Educators are a great help when you're starting a new treatment. An educator is trained to show you how to take diabetes pills, start insulin therapy, and test your blood sugar.

◆ An educator can help you stay up-to-date on the latest research and treatments (they do change frequently). Is an insulin pump a good choice for you? Could you benefit from a new oral hypoglycemic? What's a good way to fight off low blood sugar in the night? These are all good questions to pose to your educator.

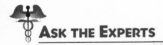

ASK THE EXPERTS

What does a registered dietitian do?

A dietitian can help you balance your food and medicine in a manner that fits your current (or changing) lifestyle. Everyone is different, and tailoring your treatment to how you work and live will give you a much better shot at keeping your blood sugar in control. If you have concurrent conditions, a dietitian can help you work out ways to deal with these, too. Since extra weight can make diabetes (and blood pressure) harder to control, a dietitian will work to help you lose weight. In an ideal situation, a registered dietitian and diabetes educator will work together. (For more information on dietitians, see page 87.)

How often should I see a dietitian?

There's no firm rule for how often you should meet, although a yearly get-together is a good start. Your doctor or educator can help you decide when you should meet with a dietitian. If you are interested in carbohydrate counting or losing weight, it's a good idea to go ahead and make an appointment. If you find that you are having quite a few high or low blood sugar counts, a dietitian can also help identify whether your eating plan needs adjustment.

What if my insurance won't cover visits to an educator?

Often insurance will cover a visit to a diabetes educator, but policies obviously vary. In some cases, you may need a physician's referral. If the insurer still will not cover meetings with an educator, ask your physician to send a letter describing the necessity of this form of treatment. Don't give up if the insurer initially says no; keep appealing. Medicare in most states now covers outpatient diabetes self-management training and programs recognized by the ADA. The ADA Web site (**www.diabetes.org**) lists such programs in your area.

Ophthalmologist
catching eye problems early

While you're making appointments, don't forget a yearly visit to an eye doctor. If you cannot seem to remember when you had your last checkup with an ophthalmologist, try using your birthday as a natural reminder.

Ophthalmologists are physicians who can help you avoid and correct the vision problems that people with diabetes sometimes face. When you arrive for your appointment, make sure to tell your doctor that you have diabetes. The doctor will put special drops in your eyes to dilate (expand) your pupils, then look at the backs of your eyes for signs of eye disease, including disorders of the retina (diabetic retinopathy), early cataracts, and glaucoma.

See your eye doctor each year so you can be certain to catch any problems. If you do begin to have diabetes-related eye problems, your doctor may ask you to come in more often. Laser treatments for retinopathy can dramatically reduce the risk of vision loss. A yearly exam should be sufficient to catch problems with the retina early enough to treat them.

Remember that controlling your blood sugar and blood pressure are the best ways to avoid eye disease. What if you begin to have some vision problems? Try to relax—changes in your blood sugar can often cause temporary changes in your vision. If they persist, call your doctor.

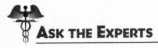

I'm really nervous about losing my vision. How likely is it?

Vision loss—this is a scary thought. Let's take a breather here. Yes, there is always a risk, but the encouraging news is that good control of blood sugar and blood pressure will dramatically reduce that risk. Moreover, laser treatment, an outpatient procedure, is a very effective way of preserving your vision.

Do I need to see an ophthalmologist or can I stick with my optometrist?

An ophthalmologist is a medical doctor who specializes in diseases of the eye. If you have diabetes, you should see one every year for a dilated-eye exam. An optometrist is not a medical doctor, but someone who is trained in examining eyes for focus problems and correcting them with glasses. (An optometrist will also look for signs of eye disease during an exam; if a problem is found, you will be referred to an ophthalmologist who will be able to medically treat your problem.)

FIRST PERSON INSIGHTS

Backup shades

I recently met with my eye doctor for my routine checkup. An assistant dilated my eyes, and then the ophthalmologist checked my eyes for signs of retinopathy. After 20 years, so far so good. The most irritating part is the paper-thin, squared-off disposable sunglasses they give you for driving home. Call me vain, but I feel ridiculous wearing them— even on the ride back to my office. I always forgot to bring sunglasses, but I finally got smart and now keep a cheap pair in my car so I won't forget.

—John F., College Park, MD

Your advocate
when you need emotional support

Diabetes is tough to handle on your own. Simply managing the disease calls for serious time-management skills, to say nothing of managing the myriad doctor appointments you will need. Add it all up and you've got a case of chronic stress from your chronic illness. (For more on this, see pages 158–159.)

You can reduce some of that stress by letting someone close to you help take some of the burden off your shoulders. That someone can be a close friend or a family member—someone who understands you and cares deeply about your well-being. What exactly can this advocate do? Consider asking your advocate to help with the following tasks:

◆ Accompanying you to your doctor appointments and perhaps bringing up a concern that you've forgotten to mention to your doctor.

◆ Preparing a healthy meal.

◆ Keeping a fast-acting sugar source on hand for low-blood-sugar moments.

◆ Exercising with you to lower stress, blood pressure, and blood sugar.

◆ Picking up supplies at the pharmacy.

◆ Lending a hand with holiday shopping.

◆ Arranging for child care when necessary.

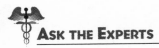

I don't want to burden my friends or family with my diabetes. Are there mental health therapists who specialize in the treatment of diabetes?

There are, in fact, therapists who treat patients with diabetes. Psychotherapy can help you develop strategies for coping with anxiety or depression that is negatively affecting your health. It's hard to take care of your diabetes when you're feeling overwhelmed. Some therapists lead support groups, and others meet one-on-one with patients or with the patient and members of the patient's family. Because diabetes can affect your personal life, you may also wish to see a couples' counselor or marriage therapist.

Ever since I was diagnosed with diabetes, my friend has not let me alone. I enjoy her help, but she goes overboard. What can I do?

It's not uncommon to find that an overly helpful friend takes on your illness as part of her problem. Let her know that while you appreciate her help, her support is backfiring. Give her specific tasks to do that will make her feel useful but will not invade your space or time. If that doesn't work, take a break from each other for a while. If the problem persists, tell her your concerns.

My brother was diagnosed with type 1 diabetes last month. He won't tell me anything about it, despite my questions. What can I do?

We all react to stress in different ways. And getting a diagnosis of a chronic illness is way up there on the stress meter. According to Dr. Shelley E. Taylor, author of *The Tending Instinct,* men and women handle certain stresses differently. Men prefer to handle emotionally stressful situations alone, confiding only in their spouses, while women prefer to share their troubles with their women friends. The thing to do is focus on activities you and your brother enjoy doing together. He will open up when he feels comfortable.

How to be a smart patient
making the most of your appointment

The door opens up in an exam room and the doctor enters and asks how you are doing. You draw a blank. All the ups and downs of the past few months seem distant and hard to remember. And it feels like the clock is ticking on your appointment.

To avoid this only-too-common situation, treat your appointment like a business meeting, complete with an agenda—in this case, a list of your questions and concerns.

Before your appointment, review your health journal (see page 22). Bring it along to help jog your memory. Be sure to bring your glucose log with you, too. If you are having difficulty with your blood sugar, it's also a good idea to write down the foods you've been eating. Note any other information that might also shed light on your situation, such as whether exercise or a later than usual meal brought on a low-blood-sugar attack. Your doctor may suggest you track your blood pressure, too. Make copies of any information you want your doctor to keep for reference.

Insurance Help

Insurance issues can be complicated and confusing if you have diabetes. It's not always clear which health services, such as meeting with a dietitian or attending a support group, will be covered. Here are some tips that can help:

◆ Call ahead to your insurance company to see if you can pre-authorize a health service, such as meeting with a diabetes educator. More and more insurance companies are realizing that covering some educational services can save them a lot of money because of the lowered risk of complications later on.

◆ Don't assume insurance won't cover a certain service. You might be surprised to find that your insurance company covers diabetes camp for children, for example, or meeting with a dietitian.

◆ Work with your doctor to get "letters of necessity" to encourage your insurance company to cover a service that the insurer initially rejects.

◆ Fill out any claim forms fully; don't provide an excuse for a rejected claim.

◆ If a claim is initially rejected, appeal it.

Support groups
you are not alone

Support groups for diabetes not only provide information and resources for people with diabetes, but also create a forum where members can share experiences and get support in a safe atmosphere. A support group can help you deal with anxieties diabetes sometimes brings on, such as changing roles for family members, feelings of lost control, and dealing with complications and the fear of them. Other common issues discussed in support groups include dealing with a new diagnosis, having difficulty with a medication, complying with diet restrictions, and general burnout.

Each support group has a facilitator who organizes the group and runs the meetings. Support groups are often led by a psychotherapist, nurse, social worker, or diabetes educator (nurse, dietitian, pharmacist, social worker, physical therapist). The facilitator can be helpful in making sure members' concerns are addressed and that medical information is accurate.

If you attend a support group, you'll likely learn about new treatments and ways to manage glucose control. You might learn about motivation techniques and how to maintain good control when you are having difficulty coping with the daily demands of diabetes. Best of all, you will be able to share your experiences and benefit from others' sharing their experiences with you.

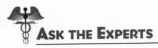

Where can I find a diabetes support group in my town?

Go online. The American Diabetes Association (**www.diabetes.org**) lists support groups by area. Or call your local hospital and ask if they know of any diabetes support groups. They are often held in hospital meeting rooms, as well as libraries, parks, churches, and community centers. If you are interested in a family support group, the Children with Diabetes Web site (**www.childrenwithdiabetes.com**) provides an excellent listing by state.

What about online support groups?

There are a number of Internet lists and newsgroups that act as support groups for people with diabetes (see pages 62-65). Online support groups work in ways similar to those of groups that meet in person—offering shared experiences, a calming voice for the newly diagnosed, and methods of reducing the stress of day-to-day living with diabetes.

I'd like to go to a support-group meeting, but the idea of speaking in front of a group makes me nervous. What can I do?

This is completely understandable and absolutely normal. Speak to the facilitator ahead of time and discuss your anxiety about attending a meeting. Bring a friend to the meeting if that makes it easier for you. Remember that a support group is designed to create a safe, comfortable space to share experiences and work through problems with people who are experiencing the same challenges you are facing.

Helpful resources

The Tending Instinct
by Shelley E. Taylor

Find a Registered Dietitian
www.cdrbet.org

Find a Diabetes Educator
**American Association of Diabetes
Educators**
www.aadenet.org

Find a Diabetes Education Program
(American Diabetes Association)
**www.diabetes.org/education/edu
state2.asp**

Eating Right

Food fundamentals
glucose and you

Most people have gone on—and off—a diet at one time or another, and if you are one of them, now is the time to get serious about it. The good news is that this doesn't mean microscopic portions or a list of foods you absolutely must avoid. You can eat most foods in moderation. What you must do is keep your blood sugar from rising too high (or falling too low if you take medication for diabetes). That's why it's important to watch the amount of carbohydrates you take in—primarily breads, cereals, pasta, rice, fruits and fruit juices, and starchy vegetables—since carbohydrates easily convert into glucose and cause blood sugar to rise.

Normally, blood glucose goes up for about two hours after you have eaten, and then drops back down. Because you have diabetes, your blood glucose does not enter cells properly and your blood sugar may remain high. Protein foods—meat, chicken, fish, cheese, eggs, soy—can also be turned into glucose, but the process is more complicated. Protein slows the absorption of carbohydrates and won't increase the need for insulin the way carbs do. That doesn't mean you should go on a low-carbohydrate, high-protein diet. In fact, this sort of diet can complicate other possible conditions, such as kidney and heart disease.

For most people, including those with diabetes, a daily diet should include six or more portions of grains, beans, and starchy vegetables and two to three servings of meat, cheese, fish, and other proteins. Fat from your diet cannot be turned into glucose; it is converted into an energy molecule called a **ketone**, but it helps keep sugar up throughout the day. Fat has about twice as many calories as similar amounts of protein and carbohydrates. Because most diabetics are also watching their weight, reducing fat in the diet can make a dramatic impact on the number of calories you're consuming.

Focus on Your Goals

You can control your diabetes and actually improve your health by focusing on a few basic goals:

1. Maintain your blood sugar at normal or near-normal levels. (You will learn how to do this by coordinating your insulin and other medications with your meals.)

2. Try to bring your blood cholesterol and blood pressure levels close to normal through a combination of diet, medication (if prescribed), and daily physical activity. Lose weight if you are overweight.

3. Create a diabetes meal plan with the help of your doctor, dietitian, or diabetes educator. Your meal plan should be easy to follow and include foods that you enjoy eating. Here are a few basics to get you started:

   ◆ Eat a wide variety of foods every day to get all the nutrients your body needs for good health. Try to include a combination of five different types of fruits and vegetables daily.

   ◆ Avoid skipping meals, which can make it more difficult to control your blood sugar.

   ◆ Watch your serving sizes. Your meal plan will include portion guidelines for each meal.

   ◆ Eat less fat. Foods that are high in certain fats can contribute to clogged blood vessels and heart disease.

   ◆ Eat fewer refined carbohydrates, such as white bread, white rice, pasta, and potatoes.

Eating for your health
how food works in your body

Food consists of three main nutrients: carbohydrates, fat, and protein. A healthy diet supplies all three, along with vitamins, minerals, and other vital compounds, such as fiber.

Carbohydrates give you energy. Grain foods, fruits, vegetables, legumes (dried peas, beans, and lentils), and dairy products all supply carbohydrates plus vitamins and minerals. Foods high in sugar, such as desserts and non-diet soft drinks, should be consumed sparingly because they supply calories without many other important nutrients. (Moreover, they will make your blood sugar soar.) High-fiber carbohydrate foods—whole-grain breads, bran cereals, legumes, vegetables, and fruits—are a wiser choice because they make you feel full, provide nutrients, and can help control your blood sugar and blood cholesterol.

Fat, found in meats, dairy products, oils, nuts, butter, and margarine, is another source of energy. Your body also uses fat to manufacture hormones. Some fats are better than others. Monounsaturated fats, found in nuts, olive oil, canola oil, and avocados, are better for your heart because they do not make blood cholesterol go up. The omega-3 fatty acids in sardines, salmon, and other fatty fish are also heart-healthy. Polyunsaturated fat, in vegetable oils like corn oil and safflower oil, is the next healthiest. Saturated fat, found in higher-fat meat and regular dairy products, and trans fat, in crackers, cookies, and commercial fried foods, should be limited. Since all fats supply a lot of calories, it's best not to eat too much of any of them.

Protein helps maintain muscles and organs in the body. Your diet should include modest portions of protein foods, such as meats, poultry, fish, dairy products, nuts, eggs, and legumes. If your blood sugar is difficult to control, your dietitian may recommend that you eat more protein and fat and fewer portions of carbohydrate foods.

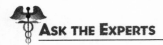

ASK THE EXPERTS

How do I find a diet that matches my lifestyle?

Personal nutritionists and dietitians are all the rage among celebrities these days. So why not one for you, especially since you have a medical reason to hire one to teach you about the basics of healthful eating and about making specific changes for diabetes? The best person to hire is a registered dietitian (R.D.) who also is a certified diabetes educator (C.D.E). The services of an R.D. for diabetes management are covered by Medicare and may be covered by your insurance company.

What is the difference between a nutritionist and a registered dietitian?

A nutritionist has studied nutrition and has often received a master's degree. Registered dietitians are health professionals who have completed an accredited education and training program and who have passed a national credentialing exam. Many registered dietitians also have master's degrees in nutrition.

How do I find a dietitian?

Your doctor will probably refer you to a registered dietitian he or she recommends for patients with diabetes. Or you can find a dietitian on your own through the Yellow Pages, by contacting the American Dietetic Association (visit **www.eatright.org** or call 800-877-1600, ext. 5000, for the names of dietitians in your area), or by asking your insurance carrier for names of approved providers.

What happens when I see a registered dietitian?

At your first appointment, your registered dietitian will review your medical history, ask questions about your current diet, and plan changes to your eating habits that are appropriate for you. At follow-up appointments, your progress will be reviewed and your diet adjusted as needed for your condition to help you reach your blood sugar and weight goals.

Hyperglycemia
when your blood sugar is too high

You're not alone if you find it difficult to keep your blood sugar level from spiking. The struggle against **hyperglycemia** (high blood sugar) is one thing people with diabetes know all too well. It's not easy to practice tight glucose control. If you find that you have frequent high blood sugar levels, you may be very uncomfortable. On the other hand, many people have no symptoms when their blood sugar is too high, which means that it goes ignored.

Here are a few of the reasons you might experience high blood sugar:

◆ You eat too much at a meal.

◆ It's the weekend. You sleep in and get a late start on your first insulin dose of the day. Your body keeps producing glucose, but there's not enough insulin in your bloodstream to help the glucose get into your cells.

◆ Your blood sugar is already elevated and you begin exercising, so your liver kicks stored glucose into your bloodstream to feed your cells with energy.

◆ You have an infection or other illness. In some cases, you might see your blood sugar rise unpredictably, before you are even aware of the illness (see pages 134–135 for more on this problem).

◆ Stress is making you anxious, which can make blood sugar rise.

◆ You have low blood sugar, and your liver releases glucose to correct the situation. This effect is sometimes called a **rebound**.

It's frustrating to check your blood sugar and see a number that's uncomfortably high. So, what can you do about it? Testing your blood glucose more often will help. Take your insulin or diabetes pills as prescribed. Regular exercise can help keep blood sugars from spiking.

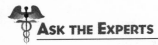
ASK THE EXPERTS

I get my hemoglobin A₁c test every few months. Isn't that enough?

While you are generally considered to be doing a good job if your glycated hemoglobin is below 7 percent, daily testing is still crucial. Remember that a glycated hemoglobin test, such as the hemoglobin A₁c, gives you an average of your blood sugar level over about 12 weeks. But it doesn't give you an immediate read on how your treatment plan is working. Also, since the test is an average, a mix of very high and very low blood sugar can make the results appear normal when, in fact, your control is all over the map.

What can I do to help correct high blood sugar?

If your blood sugar is high, drink lots of water, which can help the glucose pass through your system. If you take insulin, your doctor will help you determine how to reduce your blood sugar with a small dose of extra insulin. Don't overreact and load up on insulin, however, or you will end up with the opposite problem, unexpectedly low blood sugar.

What is ketoacidosis?

Untreated hyperglycemia in type 1 diabetes can lead to **ketoacidosis,** a condition in which the body begins burning ketones for energy instead of glucose. What are ketones? They are normal by-products your body creates when it metabolizes fats. The problem is that certain toxic acids are released when ketones instead of glucose are burned for energy. If there are too many ketones in the blood, these acids can collect in the blood; if the condition is left untreated, it can lead to coma. When your blood sugar rises above 250 mg/dl, it's important to check your urine for the presence of ketones using a ketone-testing strip. The strips are inexpensive and available at most pharmacies.

Hypoglycemia
when your blood sugar is too low

Diabetes might be called the Goldilocks Disease. You have to keep your blood sugar neither too high, as in hyperglycemia, nor too low, a condition called hypoglycemia. Low blood sugar is also called an insulin reaction. It occurs when you've taken too much insulin or your diabetes pills are kicking in and there's not enough sugar in your blood. It can make you feel weak, sweaty, and jittery, among other symptoms, and if you don't eat something quickly, you could even lose consciousness.

Hypoglycemic reactions are one of the trickier aspects of having diabetes, and they can happen unexpectedly. You may have a hypoglycemic reaction when you exercise vigorously without eating beforehand, when you take your medication and delay eating, or when you don't eat enough to cover the insulin or diabetes pills you've taken.

So what can you do about hypoglycemia? First, always keep plenty of fast-acting sugar nearby. Glucose tablets and glucose gel tend to be your best bets because they break down faster than table sugar and they don't contain a lot of unnecessary calories. Juice, candies, or a regular soda can all do the trick in a pinch. You want something with about 15 grams of fast-acting carbohydrates.

After you've treated your hypoglycemia, check your blood sugar 15 to 20 minutes later. If your blood sugar is still too low, make sure to treat it again with glucose tablets or other handy fast-acting sugar.

If you are having frequent hypoglycemic reactions, you should speak with your doctor. You may need to check your blood sugar more often. If you take insulin, make sure to eat directly after taking fast-acting insulin. And when eating out, wait until the food is in sight before taking anything that will lower your blood sugar.

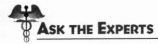

I often have low-blood-sugar reactions during the night. What can I do about them?

Hypoglycemia when you're sleeping can be scary, and dangerous. Be sure to talk to your doctor about any unusual readings; you may need an adjustment in your medication or insulin regimen. For problems at night, it's a good idea to keep some fast-acting sugar near your bed, such as glucose tablets, so you don't have to walk to the kitchen and hunt for juice or a soda when you're feeling wobbly. It's best to follow up the quick-acting sugar with a serving of carbohydrates and protein or fat to keep your blood sugar from dropping again. You might eat half a peanut butter sandwich, for example, or drink a glass of milk.

What happens if I pass out from low blood sugar?

If you are groggy or disoriented from a hypoglycemic reaction but can still swallow, the best bet is to drink a regular soda or juice, or eat a glucose gel or some other fast-acting sugar. But if you pass out from a low-blood-sugar episode, you will want to have a glucagon shot in your fridge.

Glucagon comes in a syringe preloaded with medicine that, once injected, will make your liver dump stored glucose into your bloodstream. This will make your sugar rise quickly.

Your doctor can prescribe a glucagon shot for you. The shot isn't hard to give, so it's smart to show someone in your house how to use it. The glucagon shot is injected like an insulin shot. This whole concept could be a bit scary for, say, your spouse or teenage son or daughter to deal with. Let your friends and family members know up front that giving you a glucagon shot could be a lifesaving treatment.

Using exchanges
learn how to trade foods

There's a little of the natural-born trader in all of us, and the classic tool for planning your diet cleverly takes advantage of that. The exchange system, as it's called, helps you get the nutrition you need while controlling your blood sugar. Your daily food intake is divided into a certain number of servings from the three main exchange groups, then divided into meals and snacks. Think of the exchange system like a budget: You get a certain amount of "money"—in this case, exchanges—to spend on each type of food.

Foods are grouped according to the amount of carbohydrate, protein, and fat they contain. The largest group is the Carbohydrate Group; it includes starches (bread, cereal, grain foods, and vegetables such as peas and corn), fruit, milk, nonstarchy vegetables, and other carbohydrates, such as desserts. The Meat and Meat Substitutes Group is divided into very lean, lean, medium-fat, and high-fat foods. For heart health, choose primarily from the very lean and lean lists. The Fat Group includes lists of foods with monounsaturated, polyunsaturated, saturated, and trans fats. All fats are high in calories; as such, they should be limited.

Each meal should contain one or two servings from each group—for instance, one meat and one grain food, perhaps a slice of bread with a small pat of butter, as your allowance of fat. The idea is that so long as you eat the recommended portion sizes, you will be getting a healthy—and not too large—amount of each, and not too much of any one group. You can also exchange servings within each group—say a serving of peas instead of a slice of bread or a cup of low-fat cottage cheese instead of meat. Or you might have a slice of pizza and get all three groups. The point is, you get to decide. Your dietitian will provide a long list of the permitted exchanges.

Exchange Lists vs. the Food Pyramid

Does the diabetic exchange diet plan conflict with the government's Food Guide Pyramid? Not at all. In fact, the two are very similar. Each recommends that a healthy daily diet include:

◆ 3 servings of vegetables, including starchy vegetables

◆ 2 servings of fruit

◆ 2 servings of low-fat or fat-free milk

◆ about 6 ounces of meat or meat substitutes, including beans

◆ small amounts of fat and sugar

Unlike the standard pyramid, the diabetes exchange system groups grains, beans, and starchy vegetables together because they supply similar amounts of carbohydrates per serving. (A diabetes pyramid has been developed.) Both the exchange system and the pyramid recommend selecting whole-grain foods as part of your diet.

Here's a sample of foods and portions on the diabetes Starch List:

Bagel	1/4
Bread	1 slice
Cereal, bran	1/2 cup
Corn tortilla	1
Corn, peas or potato	1/2 cup
Saltine-type cracker	6
Legumes, cooked	1/2 cup

Counting carbohydrates
a flexible eating plan

Not so many years ago, people with diabetes who took insulin had to eat
the same amount of food at about the same time every day. This made for a
simple system that helped to keep blood sugar in the normal range, but
many people had difficulty sticking to such a strict regimen and wound up
with blood sugar that was consistently too high. Carbohydrate counting,
introduced widely in the mid-1990s, can help you control blood sugar by
tying carbs to insulin intake on a sliding scale.

Counting carbohydrates gives you more flexibility in choosing foods—a
casserole, perhaps, with mixed ingredients—while still controlling your
blood sugar. The concept is fairly basic: You count the carbs in every food
that you eat (you will get booklets that tell you the exact amount of carbohydrates in most foods), measure your blood sugar about two hours after
each meal, and adjust your medication as advised by your doctor. If you
have type 1 diabetes, you will be started on a regimen of one unit of insulin
for every 15 grams of carbohydrate. Your doctor, dietitian, or diabetes educator will give you a carbohydrate goal for the day and for each meal, along
with a blood sugar goal. Your carbohydrate goal will be written as a number
of "Carb Choices," with each choice supplying 15 grams of carbohydrate. For
example, you may have three carb choices for breakfast. Each of these foods
is one carb choice: 3/4 cup unsweetened breakfast cereal, 3/4 cup blueberries,
a cup of low-fat milk. Once you know how to count carbs, your meal choices are virtually endless and your blood sugar will be much easier to control.
As you become more experienced, your diabetes educator or doctor can
help you fine-tune how many carbs will require a unit of insulin.

Because amounts and types of carbohydrate foods will affect how high
your blood sugar goes, you need to keep track of exactly what and how
much you eat. Keep a daily log of your results in your health journal (see
pages 22–23)—it will be invaluable when you meet with your doctor.

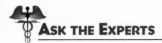

ASK THE EXPERTS

Do sweet foods affect type 1 and type 2 diabetes differently?

Sweet foods affect both types of diabetes the same way. Your insulin schedule is what regulates the way your body processes sugary desserts and candies and other carbohydrates. Don't forget any sweets—those carbohydrates should be counted in your daily total of carbohydrates or exchanges.

What is the glycemic index, and should I avoid foods with a high glycemic index?

The glycemic index (GI) measures how high your blood sugar is likely to go after eating a particular food. In general, high-fiber foods, such as oatmeal or whole-wheat bread, have a lower GI than do processed lower-fiber foods like white bread. Sugar, however, has a lower GI than do many other foods. The GI is not very useful for planning your diet.

If I'm counting carbohydrates, do I need to worry about how much protein and fat I eat?

While protein and fat do not have much effect on your blood sugar, they do supply calories. Every calorie counts if you are trying to lose weight (and losing weight can help lower your blood sugar). Eating protein, fat, and carbohydrate foods together can also cause a slower rise in your blood sugar. Keep a good food and blood-sugar record to learn how particular food combinations affect your blood sugar.

How can I count carbs when I'm eating in a restaurant?

After a while of carb counting, you get a sense of how to estimate the portions. Checking your blood sugar two hours after eating can help you see how accurate your estimate was. The big fast-food chain restaurants actually post the nutritional information (including carb count) on the wall of the restaurant or in a pamphlet you can request.

Smart food shopping
reading the label

Almost all food packages display two important sections, the Nutrition Facts panel and the Ingredient List. The Nutrition Facts panel gives amounts per serving of several nutrients that are important to people with diabetes: calories, total fat, saturated fat, sodium, and carbohydrates. The label also lists "sugars," a category that includes natural sugars, such as lactose in milk, and added sugars. You may be surprised to learn that the sugars number is not very useful to you because people with diabetes no longer have to eliminate foods with sugars. It is more important to look at calories and total carbohydrates per serving and to fit the food into your food plan.

The Ingredient List tells you which ingredients are in a particular food, from highest to lowest amounts. If sweeteners (sugar, brown sugar, evaporated cane juice, honey, molasses, high fructose corn syrup) or fats (butter, margarine, shortening, oil) appear first on the list, chances are that the food is rich in calories but not in nutrition.

Also, when you shop for food at the grocery store, keep in mind that some "diet" products can still raise your blood sugar. Low-fat salad dressings, for example, sometimes trade fat for sugar. Check out the nutritional information on foods that, at first blush, appear to be helpful to your diabetes control.

Great recipes

If you don't have a recipe book handy, the Web can help. The Diabetic Gourmet site (**www.diabeticgourmet.com**) offers hundreds of recipes that typically take less than half an hour to prepare. Each recipe includes nutritional information, such as carbohydrates, protein, fat, and calories. The American Diabetes Association also provides quick and tasty recipes on the organization's Web site, including a recipe of the day, with nutritional information (including exchanges).

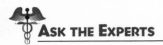

Are frozen dinners okay?

Frozen dinners are an option, especially those that are calorie-, sodium-, and portion-controlled. Many brands list diabetic exchanges and other nutritional information not usually found on food packages. Depending on your diet, you may need to include other foods to make a complete meal. Note: Most prepared foods are often very high in sodium, which can be a problem for those with high blood pressure or kidney disease.

About Sweeteners

As a person with diabetes, you have plenty of alternatives to sugar; almost all have no effect on blood sugar:

Saccharin (Sweet 'N Low™) is among the oldest sweeteners and can be used in hot or cold foods. It has a slightly bitter aftertaste.

Acesulfame potassium (acesulfame-K) retains its sweetness in cooked and baked foods. Choose recipes designed for this sweetener, as it does not have the same texture and properties as sugar.

Sucralose (Splenda™) can be used in cold or hot beverages or foods. Like other sweeteners, sucralose doesn't have the same physical properties as sugar.

Sorbitol, xylitol, and mannitol are sugar alcohols used mainly in gums and candies. They have a slight effect on blood sugar.

Aspartame (Equal™, NutraSweet™) is a strong sweetener that works best in cold foods and drinks. It contains an amino acid that should be avoided by people with a rare disorder called phenylketonuria (PKU).

All about alcohol
dealing with temptations

"Eat, drink, and be merry" is actually good advice for those who choose to consume alcohol. People with diabetes can drink alcohol in moderation, so long as they do so cautiously and have something to eat at the same time. Pure alcohol lowers blood sugar for up to 12 hours. Eating helps prevent hypoglycemia. You should also monitor your blood sugar for several hours after drinking alcohol and check it again before you go to bed. Eat a snack if your blood sugar is low.

Alternatively, some types of alcoholic beverages, namely beer, sweet wine, and drinks made with fruit juice or regular soft drinks, can make your blood sugar go up because they contain carbohydrates. Include their carbohydrate count in your daily total, or count each drink as at least one Other Carbohydrate exchange. Alcoholic drinks are not counted in the exchange system. Men who have diabetes are advised to limit themselves to two drinks per day, while women should have only one. Dilute your drink with a calorie-free mixer. Avoid alcohol if your blood sugar is not under control or if you have high blood pressure. Drinking can raise the risk of stroke and heart disease.

Mind you, that is sometimes easier said than done. Many people, when they are first diagnosed with diabetes, vow to follow exactly whatever regimen is recommended to them. But for some, that resolve fades away after a few months. What to do? The first thing is to separate the diabetes from bad habits regarding alcohol. Remember, this is not the time to be judgmental. Meet with your diabetes educator. He or she will help you identify the triggers—a stressful day, a gathering with your office buddies, a family celebration, an argument—that cause you to drink. Then he or she will help you put in "blocks": a filling snack or a nonalcoholic drink. Once the alcohol habits are under control, you can work with your educator to identify and deal with other triggers that interfere with your following your long-term diabetes regimen.

When you have a drink, your liver goes to work metabolizing the alcohol, which it treats as a toxin. In addition to breaking down alcohol, the liver is also responsible for converting stored carbohydrates to glucose. This works to keep you from getting low blood sugar, but you can find yourself with a dramatic low blood sugar when your liver is working the alcohol out of your system. So it's best to have drinks only at mealtimes and to keep an eye out for hypoglycemia.

Watching Calories and Carbohydrates

What's in a Drink?

A 150-pound person breaks down one drink in about two hours. So what do we consider "a drink"?

- 12 ounces of regular beer (150 calories)
- 5 ounces of wine (100 calories)
- 1 1/2 ounces of 80-proof distilled spirits (100 calories)

Drink Amount	Calories	Carbohydrates
Light beer 12 fl. oz.	100	5
Regular beer 12 fl. oz.	150	13
Nonalcoholic beer 12 fl. oz.	60	12
Dry wine 4 fl. oz.	80–85	0–2
Sweet wine 4 fl. oz.	105	6–7
Nonalcoholic wine 4 fl. oz.	25–35	6–7
Wine cooler 12 fl. oz.	215	30
Gin, rum, vodka, whiskey, brandy 1.5 fl. oz.	100	0
Liqueurs, cordials 1.5 fl. oz.	160	18
Bloody Mary 5 fl. oz.	115	5

Sources: American Diabetes Association and American Dietetic Association

Eating on the go
plan ahead

Anyone who has flown in recent years knows that traveling for work or pleasure can be a challenge when you have diabetes. Airplane or train meal service, even if available, may not mesh with your schedule. Food choices aloft are often limited, to put it kindly, and tight connections can put your meal- and snack-times off schedule.

For long flights, you can request special meals when you make your reservation. But for shorter flights and eating on the run, consider learning carbohydrate counting. It increases your food options and makes blood sugar control a bit easier. Work with your doctor, dietitian, or diabetes educator on a travel meal and insulin schedule, especially when you're traveling to a different time zone.

Always carry a meal, snacks, and a travel alarm. Even if you are driving, food establishments may be far off the road. Avoid sleeping through scheduled meals. Be extra aware of signs of hypoglycemia, and always carry a juice box or food to treat low blood sugar. Even at the best of times, travel can make you feel lousy, so when in doubt, check your blood sugar. This means you should always bring extra testing supplies with you, too.

Look for restaurants that offer foods you're familiar with to make it easier for you to put together meals that match your diet. Always ask how foods are prepared and how large a portion is. You may want to request a smaller portion or fill out your meal with additional side dishes to replicate your eating plan at home.

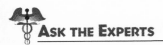

Ask the Experts

What should I do if I get sick when I'm traveling?

Diarrhea or vomiting can lead to hypoglycemia, and a fever can cause hyperglycemia. Reactions to food and colds and other ailments are tough enough when you are at home, let alone when you are away and off your regular schedule. While you are ill, check your blood sugar every two hours. If you cannot keep food down, you may need to go to the emergency room to get intravenous fluids, including glucose.

Is it okay to eat fast food on a regular basis?

Traditional fast-food burgers, fried chicken, fries, and breakfast sandwiches are high in fat and saturated fat, making them poor choices for heart and overall health. A McDonald's Big Mac, for example, has 590 calories and 34 grams of fat and 47 grams of carbs. The good news is that many fast-food chains now offer salads, grilled chicken, fruit, and other foods that fit into a healthful diabetic diet. Of course, you should choose foods that best fit into your eating pattern for that particular meal.

About caffeine

Caffeine does not affect blood sugar in most people. But the other things you put in your coffee or tea can do so, and you need to factor milk and other creamers (and sugar or honey) into your daily totals. And just in case you are one of the minority who are affected by caffeine, check your blood sugar carefully on days when you get more caffeine than usual. The symptoms of excess caffeine—jitters, headaches, nervousness, anxiety—resemble hypoglycemia and can mask its warning signs. If you choose to cut down on caffeine, switch to decaf coffee or tea, or try herbal teas.

Diabetes at all ages
handling food issues for all needs

Diabetes and Children

Children with diabetes need to live as normal a life as possible. Primary goals (in addition to blood sugar control) are to create insulin routines that work for meals and activities and to ensure that children with diabetes get the calories and nutrients they need for normal growth. Type 2 diabetes is increasingly common in children because of its relationship to obesity and weight problems. Children who "grow into" their weight—that is, get taller without gaining weight—may even outgrow type 2 diabetes. Advise your child's school, child-care provider, and friends' parents of your child's food and insulin schedule so that they know the proper way to feed your child.

Diabetes and Teens

It's doubly, even triply, tough being a teen with diabetes and having to keep blood sugar steady while dealing with hormonal changes and fitting in with friends. Teens need to monitor blood sugar regularly and be taught how to make diet changes accordingly. Encourage healthful eating by serving such high-fiber foods as whole-grain bread or cereal, beans, and popcorn, stocking up on cut vegetables and fruit in the fridge, and serving small portions of dessert on occasion. Help your child manage blood sugar during after-school physical activities. If possible, his or her blood sugar should be checked prior to exercise. Exercise should be avoided if blood sugar levels are too low, and meals should never be skipped. Explore with your teen the menus at popular restaurants and help identify the "safest" meals and snacks to order when they are out with friends.

Diabetes and Pregnancy

About 4 percent of pregnant women develop diabetes during pregnancy, even though their blood sugar had previously been normal. Your doctor, dietitian, and diabetes educator will work with you to develop a meal, exercise, and medication plan to help keep your blood sugar under control during pregnancy. Women with gestational diabetes are more likely to develop type 2 diabetes later in life, so take preventive measures after your pregnancy: Lose any extra weight you gained. Eat plenty of fruits and vegetables. Find activities that you like and that fit your daily routine, such as walking, mother-and-baby exercise classes, or swimming.

Diabetes and the Older Adult

Work with a registered dietitian to develop an eating plan that helps control blood sugar and meets nutritional needs. Older adults require fewer calories and may not be able to get enough physical activity to boost calorie burning. That is why every bite has to count toward supplying both calories and essential vitamins and minerals. If possible, prepare single-portion meals or entrées that can be frozen and heated up as needed. Purchase fresh fruits and vegetables in season. Buy only enough food for the next few days, or divide your purchases and freeze them into smaller portions. For example, berries can be washed, dried, and frozen; packages of chicken can be split into single servings; potatoes can be mashed and frozen in small portions.

FIRST PERSON INSIGHTS

Let me eat cake!

Nothing aggravates me more than when my friends tell me how to eat. After I mentioned my diabetes to one dear friend, she started making comments about what I ate whenever we met for lunch. The last time we got together, I ordered cake. She all but screamed at me. I was so mad I told her to mind her own business. Then she burst into tears! I had to explain that even though I have diabetes I can still eat sugar every now and then in moderation. I can adjust for the cake with extra insulin later. She hasn't said a word about my diet choices since.

—Anne T., Niagara Falls, NY

Helpful resources

*The Complete Guide to
Carbohydrate Counting*
by Hope S. Warshaw and
Karmeen Kulkarni
This book is the A to Z guide to carbohydrate counting for people with
diabetes.

*The Diabetes Food and Nutrition
Bible: A Complete Guide to
Planning, Shopping, Cooking, and
Eating*
by Hope S. Warshaw, Robyn Webb,
and Graham Kerr
Nutrition guidelines, menu planner,
and cookbook that teach you how to
shop, plan nutritious meals, and
cook low-fat and healthy foods.

*Diabetes Meal Planning Made Easy:
How to Put the Food Pyramid to
Work for Your Busy Lifestyle*
by Hope S. Warshaw
The Diabetes Food Pyramid helps
make meal planning easy. Learn
how to make smart food choices at
home and in the supermarket.

Eat Out, Eat Right!
by Hope S. Warshaw
This book is an updated guide to
eating in ethnic restaurants and
when traveling.

Express Lane Diabetic Cooking
by Robyn Webb
Enjoy more than 150 recipes made
with ingredients from the deli,
frozen-food, and salad-bar sections
of the grocery store.

*Guide to Healthy Restaurant
Eating, 2nd Edition*
by Hope S. Warshaw
This guide includes essential nutrition facts for more than 3,500 menu
items from nearly 60 major restaurant chains.

*Mr. Food's Quick & Easy Diabetic
Cooking*
by Art Ginsburg
More than 150 classic recipes with
nutritional information and diabetic
exchanges.

*The New Family Cookbook for
People with Diabetes*
American Diabetes Association and
American Dietetic Association
This book contains more than 400
easy recipes, along with the basics of
a diet for diabetes.

**American Association of Diabetes
Educators**
www.diabeteseducator.org
The site offers information on diabetes, links to organizations and
product information, and referrals
to certified diabetes educators
(C.D.E.'s).

CHAPTER 6

Complementary *Therapies*

Weighing your alternatives
identifying your needs

For some people, living with a chronic illness is the first time they have ever taken their health seriously enough to reflect on their lifestyle and make changes. For others, there is only anger at symptom flare-ups and the feeling of being at the mercy of the unknown. Somewhere in between lies a happy medium—a place for symptom relief and a restored sense of well-being. Enter the world of complementary medicine.

What will work for you depends on what troubles you most about your illness. If you are frightened or angry or depressed, you may benefit from techniques that emphasize the mind-body connection, such as biofeedback, meditation, and psychotherapy, or from exercise that requires mental focus, such as yoga or tai chi. On the other hand, some people find that this kind of mental retraining increases their stress and they prefer to treat these symptoms within the strict guidelines of traditional medicine.

Complementary therapies are often called "alternative medicine." But to call something an "alternative" suggests that you do either one or the other. It's more useful and more accurate to think of these treatments as supplemental or complementary to your standard medical treatment. As you explore complementary therapies, be certain to discuss your plans and discoveries with your doctor, not only because it's essential that he or she knows what you are doing and how it might interact with your standard treatment but also because what helps you might help others.

◆ **Research what's available.** Support groups can be extremely helpful sources of information. Ask the research librarian at your library to help you. Do an Internet search using the name of your illness + the name of the therapy you want to explore. (For more information on using the Internet, see pages 45–66.)

◆ **Avoid thinking that because something is "natural," it is benign.** Many of the so-called natural substances touted by alternative healers have not been tested, let alone approved, by the FDA. Anecdotal evidence does not make it "safe." Be especially wary of taking any products that are sold directly by a healer. Talk with your doctor first before you try anything.

◆ **Stay alert to how you are feeling.** It's tempting to think that you "feel lousy all the time." In truth, you probably have good days and bad days. The more you know about what makes you feel better or worse, the more you can use that knowledge to improve your well-being. Review your health journal (see page 22).

◆ **Bear the expense in mind.** Complementary treatments can cost as much as standard methods—or more, given that many are not covered by insurance plans. Be as frank about your finances as you are about your physical condition. Some practitioners may be willing to negotiate their fees.

◆ **Above all, do not fall for the notion that if the therapy fails, you have failed.** Nothing, not even antibiotics, works equally well for everyone. Give the new therapy a fair trial—some can take a while to show a benefit—but if you are not being helped, give it up and try something else. Or talk to another person who practices the same therapy; that person may have an insight that makes all the difference.

Massage & bodywork
the lowdown on getting a rubdown

The stress response can easily cause our muscles to tighten. Not surprisingly, chronic stress can lead to chronic muscle fatigue and pain. One way to mitigate the stress in your life is through bodywork. *Bodywork* is the catchall word for a range of physical therapies that involve manipulation of the body. As with other complementary therapies, bodywork is very helpful at relieving stress-related symptoms.

People who practice therapeutic massage generally avoid the words *masseuse* and *masseur* and instead call themselves "massage therapists." Their ads will state that they practice therapeutic, medical, or sports massage; in states where the practice is regulated by the government, the abbreviation LMT (licensed massage therapist) may follow the person's name. Another string of letters to look for is NCTMB. This means that the therapist has received at least 500 hours of training and has passed a qualifying exam administered by the National Certification Board for Therapeutic Massage and Bodywork. In states where massage is a licensed health practice, your insurance company may reimburse some of the costs.

In general, *massage* means Swedish and/or Shiatsu massage and *bodywork* encompasses a wide range of other physically based therapies. Another distinction, albeit a fine one, is that massage is often limited to physical manipulation and bodywork encompasses the idea that the body is also composed of energy fields and channels and that blocked energy causes or exacerbates disease.

The different practices vary in intensity and therapeutic benefits; almost all of them can be successfully administered while you are clothed. Also, different therapists have different "touches"—some work gently, others work vigorously. Ask the therapist how much discomfort you might experience as an inherent part of the treatment, and if the therapist is working too deeply, speak up.

Here's a look at some popular bodywork therapies. To get more information or for help in locating a practitioner, see Helpful Resources, page 118.

Swedish massage Originally intended to help improve blood circulation and encourage drainage of the lymph system, this technique uses gliding, kneading, tapping, or vibrating strokes for gentle or penetrating muscle massage. It is especially helpful for tension relief and relaxation.

Myofascial therapy This is a general term for a number of techniques that manipulate soft tissue—*myo-*, muscle fibers, and *fascia*, the connective tissue that holds muscle fibers in place—to relieve "trigger points," localized areas that are painful themselves or provoke pain in other areas.

Rolfing Developed by Ida P. Rolf, a biochemist who called the process "Structural Integration," it is a form of deep manipulation of the body's soft tissues to balance energy and relieve chronic pain and stress. Practitioners are trained and certified by the Rolf Institute, in Colorado.

Shiatsu (acupressure) A component of traditional Chinese medicine. Practitioners use fingertip pressure on specific points along the body's energy channels to release blocks, restore balance, and encourage health.

Craniosacral Therapy (CST) Developed by an osteopath, Dr. John E. Upledger. Practitioners gently manipulate the skull, the sacrum, and the nerve endings in the scalp. It is helpful for back and neck pain, headache, sinus infections, stress and tension, chronic fatigue, and fibromyalgia. Practitioners are trained and certified by the Upledger Institute, in Florida.

The Trager Approach Nonintrusive massage and movement reeducation focusing on integrating the mind and body to relieve anxiety. Practitioners are trained and certified by the Trager Institute, in Ohio.

Stress management
teaching your mind to soothe your body

Stress can make your blood sugar and blood pressure rise and trigger the body's fight-or-flight response, which releases hormones that make insulin less efficient. Even when you're no longer under stress, your body can produce hormones that will affect your blood sugar control. Stored glucose is released into the bloodstream when you are stressed and you might not have enough insulin to keep up. Even worse, stress increases the risk of hypertension, heart attacks, strokes, and damage to the kidneys.

Learning to relax sounds counterintuitive, even insultingly simplistic. Relaxing should be instinctive and, under most circumstances, it is. But being diagnosed with a chronic illness is a life-changing, anxiety-provoking experience and it's easy to get so bound up with stress that you don't realize how stressed you are. Practitioners of the so-called mind-body modalities teach you to be more conscious of stress and give you practical things to do about it. Again, it may seem counterintuitive to focus on stress—after all, we're hardwired to recoil from pain and culturally programmed to pull up our socks and get on with things. But with proper guidance, stress management can yield enormous benefits, not just physically but also mentally, emotionally, and spiritually. When you feel better, you are better.

Biofeedback was one of the earliest stress-management techniques to gain credence with medical doctors, perhaps because it uses computers to audit measurable physiological functions. In a typical session, you may have a few small sensors attached to your head, your hands (or just a finger), or your heart. The sensors measure your brain waves, skin temperature, heart rate, level of muscle tension, and blood pressure. These sensors are connected to a computer that displays this information in graph form on a computer screen or converts it to a specific sound you can hear through the computer's speakers. As you watch the screen, you can see your heart rate slowing and your muscles relaxing. As you do this, your heart rate will even out and your muscles will relax. This improves blood flow, which raises the temperature in your hands. The computer screen gives you ongoing visual and auditory feedback about your physical condition. You can actually see how changing your mind changes your body. People usually need about 12 sessions to master the technique. Imagine learning how to calm your racing heart simply by using your mind. Because of its clinical effectiveness, the National Institutes of Health considers biofeedback an underutilized therapy. You might want to check it out and see if it can help.

Relaxation therapy encompasses a wide range of techniques designed to reduce stress and tension. Some of the more popular ones are:

Progressive muscle relaxation You do this by systematically tensing and relaxing the muscles in each part of your body. While sitting comfortably or lying down, inhale and clench your facial muscles, hold the tension for a moment, then exhale and relax those muscles. Do the same thing with your shoulders, one arm, then the other—and so on through your body until you get to your toes. When you are done, stay quietly where you are and breathe normally for a few minutes.

Guided imagery The idea here is to imagine a peaceful place and put yourself in the scene. This is usually done with a partner who provides the "guidance" by describing the scene, but you can do all the imagining yourself or listen to a narrated audiotape or to soothing music or environmental sounds, such as birdsong or ocean waves.

Diaphragmatic breathing Taking a few minutes each day to practice slow, deep breathing can relieve muscle pain and light-headedness and improve mental acuity. All you need to do is stand, sit, or lie still; slowly inhale until you feel your lungs pressing against your stomach; then exhale slowly and completely. Repeat for 10 or 12 breaths, and try to do this from time to time throughout the day. Some people find it energizing to do before they get out of bed in the morning.

Meditation
using the metaphysical to help the physical

Studies show that regular meditation can lower blood pressure, relieve chronic pain, and reduce cortisol levels, a measure of the body's stress. It may also help if you suffer from frequent and severe headaches. It can also help teach your body how to relax. Dr. Herbert Benson, a cardiologist, did a great deal of research on meditation and found that it can actually lower autonomic nervous system activity. Meaning, meditation allows your body to truly relax. Dr. Benson dubbed this phenomenon "the relaxation response."

How can something so simple work such wonders? There is no hard answer. Most practitioners say it works because it brings both the body and the mind into a uniquely unified state. As Dr. Lawrence Edwards, a meditation teacher in Bedford Hills, New York, explains, "Meditation is a transformation process. Over time, meditation profoundly changes the mind and the body, allowing you to more quickly access a state of peace and inner freedom. Every time you meditate, you are increasing the reservoir of meditative power that you can tap into during stressful or challenging moments."

There are a number of different meditation techniques to consider. Some focus on the breath, simply observing yourself breathing in and out; others use a mantra (a sacred word or phrase) that you repeat over and over again. The goal is the same: to focus your attention away from the thoughts whirling around inside your head. The repetition of breath or mantra helps calm down the mind so it can enter into a meditative state. Unlike guided imagery (see page 111), classic meditation does not involve talking or music, but it may be helpful to light a scented candle or burn incense. That's because your mind will associate the fragrance with "it's time to settle down," and that can help ease your transition into the practice. It's also helpful to meditate at the same time every day and for the same amount of time.

How to Meditate

Find a place you can sit quietly without interruption for 20 minutes.

Sit comfortably, but keep your back erect—this will help promote alertness and open breathing. (You can meditate lying down, if you are not able to sit up.)

Set a timer for 15 to 20 minutes.

Close your eyes and bring your attention to your breathing. Focus on the movement of your diaphragm as you inhale and exhale.

As you settle into this quiet breathing, you can repeat your mantra or any word you wish silently to yourself. You can use the traditional Sanskrit words *Om Namah Shivaya*, silently repeat a phrase of your own choosing, or simply use the words "one, two, three, four."

When your mind begins to wander, as it inevitably will, just gently return your focus to your breath or mantra. This pattern of wandering and returning is the beginning of teaching your mind to let go of its worries.

When the timer buzzes, notice how at peace you feel. Open your eyes and stretch.

Choose a regular time and place to meditate. Start by meditating for 20 minutes three times a week. Stay with it.

Yoga, the "mindful" exercise
using yoga to help your diabetes

The goals of yogic exercise are to teach you to pay attention to your body as you breathe and exercise. You want to coordinate your breath with your movements. For this reason, some people consider yoga a "mindful" exercise, a form of meditation in motion. But how does that help your health? Studies have shown that yoga has a strong antidepressant effect and that it promotes mental and emotional clarity; improves balance, flexibility, strength, and stamina; relieves chronic muscle aches; eliminates stress; and helps to regulate your metabolism.

There are variations in the way yoga is taught. Some classes are slow-paced, others are as lively as a step-aerobics class. Typically, yoga classes can be paid for one at a time or in sets of 5 or 10 with a discounted price. If you are curious but skeptical, ask to observe a class; you should be able to do this for free. Class lengths vary: A midday class may be 30 or 45 minutes, but an evening class may be 60 or 90 minutes long—and priced accordingly. Shop around until you find something that suits you. A number of books, videotapes, and DVDs are available that feature beginner's exercises that you can do at home.

Qigong and tai chi

According to the National Qigong Association, qigong is "an ancient Chinese health care system that integrates physical postures, breathing techniques, and focused intention." Pronounced "CHEE gung"—and sometimes spelled "Chi Kung"—the word means "cultivating energy." Tai chi is a form of qigong; both are practiced for health maintenance, healing, and increased vitality. Tai chi is also a martial art, and the sequence of gestures used in it help to prepare the person, mentally and physically, for fighting. Both qigong and tai chi consist of a specific series of dancelike gestures that are performed in a specific sequence. The sequence of gestures is called a form, and there are long and short forms of the exercises. In tai chi, the short form takes about 10 minutes to complete. It's a bit longer for qigong. Practitioners of the form say that the sense of vitality you feel afterward will last throughout the day.

FIRST PERSON INSIGHTS

Finally, help for my aching back

A friend recommended that I see a local massage therapist to alleviate some lower back pain after a day of gardening. I met the practitioner in her office and we talked a bit about my back pain and the kind of work I do throughout the day. She showed me two stretches that would help alleviate some tension. She told me she would leave the room for a few minutes so I could undress down to my underwear, lie facedown on the table, and pull the sheet over me. After a few minutes, she knocked on the door and asked if I was ready. I said yes and she came in and dimmed the lights, turned on some soothing music, and poured a bit of body oil in her hands. For the next hour, she worked on my back. Once I got over being nervous, I found myself relaxing. When she hit a troublesome spot, she asked me to breathe along with her while she worked on it. It was really amazing, and by the end of the session, my back felt great.

—Eric L., Austin, TX

Beware of quackery
avoiding marketing schemes and scams

If you spend any time researching diabetes on the Internet, you will see ads for diabetes "cures" and various herbal supplements that are said to alleviate diabetes-related health problems. These come-ons often appear on bulletin boards on Web sites and in mailing lists for people with diabetes.

Some common scams include marketing schemes that try to get you to buy weight-loss products and herbal supplements that allegedly reduce blood sugar levels, with no data to back up the claims. Somewhat scarier are claims found on the Web that suggest a cure for type 1 diabetes and offer replacements for insulin. There is, of course, no replacement for insulin. These claims are patently, knowingly false. Avoid them at all costs. If it sounds too good to be true, it probably is.

You can find more information about diabetes and quackery at the Children with Diabetes Web site, which does an excellent job of debunking common scams. You can also look up information on specific offers with a great service called Quackwatch (**www.quackwatch.com**). The site investigates claims that are questionable and answers consumers' questions on products that appear to be misleading or fraudulent.

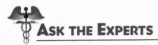
ASK THE EXPERTS

I've seen ads for chromium claiming that it lowers blood sugar. Does it work?

Chromium is a supplement that has long been promoted as a way to lower blood sugar by increasing insulin sensitivity in people with type 2 diabetes. Chromium, a mineral, is found in brewer's yeast as well as in cereals and grains. Some studies have shown that high doses of chromium, especially in people who were chromium deficient, did reduce blood sugar levels, but scientists differ on whether chromium is an effective or safe supplement. Your treatment plan of diet, exercise, and oral hypoglycemics is still the best bet for controlling type 2 diabetes.

Can high doses of vitamins alleviate symptoms of diabetes?

Again, no. Take these claims with a truckload of salt. The Internet is, sadly, brimming with these sorts of get-rich-quick schemes aimed at people with diabetes and other chronic illnesses. The people who push these products are deceitful and shameless.

Helpful resources

*Diabetes Burnout: What to Do When
You Can't Take It Anymore*
by William H. Polonsky

**National Center for
Complementary and Alternative
Medicine (NCCAM)
National Institutes of Health
Bethesda, MD 20892
Tel: 888 644-7227
http://nccam.nih.gov**
This government agency provides
information about and sponsors
research on complementary
therapies.

**American Council on Science
and Health**
1995 Broadway
New York, NY 10023-5860
**Tel: 212 362-7044
fax: 212 362-4919
www.acsh.org**

www.alternativehealing.org
This site is full of advice and explanations about every kind of alternative treatment under the sun.

www.quackwatch.com
This organization keeps tabs on
fringe alternative therapies.

Living Smart

Exercise at work and play
what you need to know

Exercise can dramatically lower your blood sugar for up to 24 hours after you engage in it. This is a great benefit, but if you have diabetes, it is a benefit that needs to be treated with some caution. Your glucose meter can help you figure out how various activities, such as housework, affect your blood sugar level. You'll get a good idea of how your body reacts by measuring your blood sugar before you mop the floor, and then an hour or two afterward. Talk to your physician about cutting back insulin or, if you don't take insulin, having a snack before any activity that makes your blood sugar drop.

You can incorporate your daily activities into an exercise regimen. If you work up a sweat chopping wood, gardening, or playing with your children or grandchildren, you are on your way to becoming fit and keeping your blood sugar in the normal range. The best activities for lowering your blood sugar level are those you enjoy and will stick with. Don't forget, chores can get your heart pumping and help you burn up as many calories as exercise.

- Here are some chores that double as exercise:
- Walking the dog
- Raking leaves
- Washing your car
- Cleaning your house

The Medical College of Wisconsin studied a group of people doing various activities while measuring their vital signs and energy expended. The results may surprise you. You can, for instance, burn 100 calories cleaning or vacuuming for 25 to 35 minutes. See the chart on the opposite page for more ideas on calorie burning.

Exercise and Chore Calorie Counting

Hate working out? You are not alone. According to the Centers for Disease Control and Prevention, you can burn 150 calories a day, or a little over 1,000 calories a week, doing the following activities:

Washing and waxing the car	45–60 minutes
Washing windows or floors	45–60 minutes
Playing volleyball	45 minutes
Playing touch football	30–45 minutes
Gardening	30–45 minutes
Wheeling self in wheelchair	30–40 minutes
Basketball (shooting baskets)	30 minutes
Bicycling 5 miles	30 minutes
Dancing fast (social)	30 minutes
Pushing a stroller 1 1/2 miles	30 minutes
Raking leaves	30 minutes
Walking 2 miles	30 minutes (15 mins/mile)
Water aerobics	30 minutes
Swimming laps	20 minutes
Wheelchair basketball	20 minutes
Basketball (playing a game)	15–20 minutes
Bicycling 4 miles	15 minutes
Jumping rope	15 minutes
Running 1 1/2 miles	15 minutes (10 mins/mile)
Shoveling snow	15 minutes
Stairwalking	15 minutes

Sex and diabetes
don't be afraid to ask questions

Sex can sometimes be a cause of anxiety for both men and women with diabetes. That's because low blood sugar can bring a romantic evening to a screeching halt, at least temporarily, while you shakily grab something with sugar to eat. And high blood sugar can make you feel lethargic, grumpy, and generally not in the mood.

For men, circulation problems can reduce the ability to have and maintain an erection, sometimes called erectile dysfunction, or impotence. Narrowing of the blood vessels can restrict blood flow to the tissue that stiffens during an erection. Nerve damage can also make having and maintaining an erection difficult.

In women, diabetes can lead to hardening of the blood vessels in the vaginal wall, causing vaginal dryness. Diabetes, in particular during menopause, can also increase the risk of yeast infections.

All these difficulties are very treatable. See your doctor. There are tests you can take to help determine the cause. For men with erectile dysfunction, a doctor might prescribe oral medicine, such as sildenafil citrate, marketed as Viagra. For women, an over-the-counter lubricant is sometimes recommended for vaginal dryness. Problems such as lack of sensitivity or difficulty with orgasm might prompt a referral to a gynecologist. There are medications that can help with low libido.

You can reduce the risk of sexual dysfunction. It's probably no surprise that tight blood sugar control can help. Reducing stress and alcohol intake also helps. In some cases, the cause of impotence may be psychological, driven by fear of the condition, even when no physical problems are present. Also, you should quit smoking, as it can restrict blood flow.

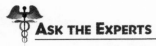

ASK THE EXPERTS

Do people with diabetes have more cases of impotence than those who don't have diabetes?

Erectile dysfunction does tend to appear in men with diabetes sooner than in the general population. But again, good blood sugar control can help. And remember that, while it's true that high blood sugar over time increases the risk of erectile dysfunction, it's a treatable condition. Close to a quarter of all men's doctor appointments in 1999 concerned the inability to have or maintain an erection, according to the National Ambulatory Medical Care Survey.

What can I do about low-blood-sugar moments during sex?

Like other physical activity, sex can make your blood sugar drop precariously. It's smart to have a snack if you know you are going to have sex, so that a low doesn't get in the way. A small snack, such as one you might eat before bedtime when your sugar is below 120 mg/dl, can be helpful. Try to eat something with a little carbohydrate (such as one serving of crackers or a piece of bread) and protein (or a small amount of fat, such as a tablespoon of peanut butter). Obviously, not all sex is planned, but a little preparation can help when you know you're going to have a romantic evening (or morning, or afternoon . . .).

Where should I put my insulin pump during sex?

You can briefly disconnect a pump for romantic moments, so check with your doctor about this and discuss how long it would be okay to be disconnected. If you'd just rather not disconnect, you can place it under a pillow or on a nightstand. It's a matter of preference.

Finding insurance
join a group

Getting insurance when you have a preexisting condition like diabetes can be difficult. Medicare covers blood-testing supplies and diabetes education for folks who are older than 65 and people who have serious diabetic complications, such as kidney disease. The real trick is obtaining inexpensive insurance if your company doesn't offer a group health insurance plan or if you are self-employed. If you need individual health insurance, as 16 million other Americans do, it's likely that you will see a surcharge for a preexisting condition or possibly be rejected by some insurers. In 2002, 46 states had laws requiring that insurers cover diabetic treatments and supplies. Sometimes you can buy insurance through an affiliate group (a lodge, for instance), a union, or a professional association.

Discrimination

You cannot be turned down for a job because of your diabetes. The Americans with Disabilities Act, passed in 1990, protects civilian employees who work for companies with more than 15 people. For example, your employer cannot ask whether you have diabetes when you are being hired. The Rehabilitation Act of 1973 and the Congressional Accountability Act protect federal employees from discrimination because of a disability in the workplace.

Some government agencies, such as the military and the FBI, have blanket bans against hiring people with diabetes. Many law-enforcement organizations do hire people with diabetes, and in the future, perhaps, they will serve in the U.S. military as individuals with diabetes do in many other countries.

Don't ignore the effect of stress

I was diagnosed with type 2 diabetes when I was 64 years old. It took a year to get my blood sugar under control. The problem was that my job as a line mechanic confined me to certain duties for long periods of time. I would often use my morning coffee break to eat my entire lunch! Then the layoffs started. We were asked to do the jobs of those laid off. I was getting really stressed, and my blood glucose levels were way out of control. I also developed a chronic sinus infection that I just could not beat. My doctor was worried because my diabetes was getting worse. He said the stress was too much and suggested I take an extended sick leave. The union was for it, but I was afraid management would boot me out. My union made a deal, and I ended up being able to retire early with full benefits. I am glad my doctor forced the issue. Another year in that situation, and who knows what would have happened.

—Tom S., Glen Burnie, MD

Eating out
blame it on pizza

When eating out, most of us don't head straight for the healthiest entrée on the menu, but instead look for an opportunity to kick back, enjoy the moment, and try new, appetizing dishes. You can certainly eat the foods you love, but it's helpful to keep a few things in mind that won't push your blood sugar to dizzying new heights.

First, don't be afraid to ask your waiter what's in the food you eat. It might take a run back to the kitchen to find out, but most servers are glad to do it. If you feel uncomfortable asking about the nutritional content of a meal—or cannot get it for some reason—look for foods that you know agree with your blood sugar. You will especially need to keep an eye on how many carbohydrates you are taking in.

So, what kinds of foods make your blood sugar spike? Your glucose meter can help you determine trends, especially if you test:

1. Just before eating
2. An hour or two after eating
3. Before bedtime

Some foods are difficult for some folks to handle. Pizza is a known culprit, because it can raise blood sugar levels for hours after eating it. Does that mean you should give it up? Certainly not—just eat it in moderation. And keep your glucose meter handy to see how any given meal is affecting your blood sugar.

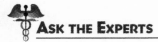

ASK THE EXPERTS

I was rushing for a dinner date and forgot my medication. Rather than going back home to get it, what else could I have done?

If you cannot make it home to pick up your medicine, here are a few tips for making the best of your situation:

1. Look for a meal, such as a salad, that goes light on the carbohydrates. Try to avoid dressings that are likely to have sugar (French, Russian, Thousand Island) and stick with a low-calorie topping, such as oil and vinegar or oil and lemon.

2. After your meal, take a long walk if you can to burn off some of the calories and keep your blood sugar level in check.

What kinds of foods should I look for in a restaurant?

Many restaurants now offer healthy menu options low in salt, calories, and fat. Salads, minus gobs of cheese and dressing, are an obvious choice. Lean meats and fish are good, especially if they are baked or grilled. Look for steamed foods, such as seafood and vegetables, that are cooked without fat. Soups can be very high in sodium, so if you're concerned about that, ask your server if the restaurant has a low-salt soup.

Which foods should I definitely avoid when eating out?

Fried foods are certainly good to avoid because they are high in fat and calories, although you can remove the breading from some fried foods to minimize the damage. Cream-based sauces are typically high in fat and calories, so a marinara sauce, for example, is often a better option. Portion control is especially important when you eat out, since menu items are probably higher in fat and salt than those you prepare at home. Share the wealth and split an entrée with a friend. Or take what you don't eat home for tomorrow's lunch.

Traveling with diabetes
crossing time zones can be tricky

When delays turn the 8 PM flight to Boston into the 12 AM red-eye, your stress level can go through the roof. And we know that stress, along with unusual mealtimes and eating on the run, can make your blood sugar hard to control. In general, it helps to check your blood sugar more often than normal while traveling.

If you have a hectic travel schedule, avoid taking your insulin or meal-time diabetes pills until just before you are served to avoid low blood sugar. Keep glucose tablets, candy, or juice with you to correct unexpected lows. Crossing time zones can be especially tricky. Talk to your physician about taking more or less medicine, depending on whether your travel will lengthen or shorten your day. As a general rule of thumb, wait until the first full day of your trip to adjust when you take your medicine and eat in a new time zone.

Preflight Checklist

"Can I take syringes on a plane? Will my glucose meter set off the X-ray machine? How do I explain an insulin pump to airport security?"

The Transportation Security Administration (TSA), established after September 11, 2001, has made provisions for those with diabetes who are flying—notably, that you need to keep your supplies with you, rather than packed away in a bag and checked onto the plane.

The policies, according to many with diabetes, are rather loosely enforced, but you should be aware of them. Here are the TSA regulations that most directly affect individuals with diabetes who need to fly: Notify the screener that you have diabetes and are carrying your supplies with you. The following supplies and equipment are allowed through the checkpoint once they have been screened: insulin (properly labeled) and insulin-loaded dispensing products such as syringes, lancets, glucose meters, test strips, and insulin pumps. When used syringes need to be in a carry-on, ensure that they are in a hard, plastic-capped container. Notify screeners if you are wearing an insulin pump and, if necessary, ask the screener to examine the pump without your having to disconnect it.

Travel tips

Bring twice as much medicine and testing strips as you'll need. The most important thing is to pack your medicine in your carry-on luggage so you won't be separated from your pills or insulin and glucose meter. Pack an extra set of medicines and strips in your checked luggage.

Bring extra prescriptions. If, for whatever reason, you find yourself without the medicine you need, you will be able to get a refill. If your pharmacy is part of a national chain, you may be able to fill a prescription in a different town—or a different state. Ask before you leave. Large pharmacy chains, such as Walgreens and CVS, can often fill prescriptions by pulling up your prescriptions in a computer and then transferring your prescription from one store to another.

When you fly or take a train, ask for a diabetic meal. These meals are typically lower in sugar, sodium, fat, and calories than the other meals served. And, while the other passengers wait patiently, you are often served more quickly when you order a special meal. Note that you will probably need to order a diabetic meal at least two days in advance.

Wear a MedicAlert bracelet. It's a good idea to have some form of identification that indicates that you have diabetes in an emergency. If you don't have one yet, now is a good time to look into it (see Helpful Resources on page 130).

Helpful resources

Diabetes Day by Day: Men's Sexual Health
by American Diabetes Association

101 Tips for Coping with Diabetes
by American Diabetes Association

Nutrition and physical-activity information
Centers for Disease Control
www.cdc.gov/nccdphp/dnpa

Diabetic Gourmet
www.diabeticgourmet.com

MedicAlert Foundation
www.medicalert.org

Transportation Security Administration (TSA)
www.tsa.gov/public

Sick Days

Dealing with flu and colds
they make your blood sugar rise

All sorts of sicknesses and stresses can increase your body's production of glucose, making you feel worse and increasing the need for insulin. It's no surprise that the virus that's going around makes you feel worse than everyone in your office, school, or house. Take heart. Yes, blood sugar will bounce around when you're sick, but it should normalize soon after your illness is gone. That said, you still need to take special care when you are sick. The problem is that when you are feeling weak or nauseated, it can be difficult to keep food down and maintain a normal blood sugar level. But it's very important to keep taking your medicine. Your illness might, in fact, increase your need for insulin.

When you are so sick that you cannot eat, low blood sugar can complicate things and make you feel even worse. Call your doctor if you cannot keep food down, and stay in close contact with your doctor's office to discuss which over-the-counter medicines you can take for your symptoms. Also call your doctor if you have a fever, as fevers can wreak havoc with your blood sugar. Your doctor can tell you whether you need to adjust your medication or not.

You can use several testing methods (see page 134) to keep yourself comfortable at home. There's no reason a cold or flu should make you worry, but there are a few things to watch out for that can make your illness easier to take.

Which Is It?

The Flu The flu, or influenza, is a respiratory infection. Common symptoms are aches, fever, headache, exhaustion, and a cough that lasts a week or more. The flu can be very serious if you're are an individual with diabetes. In fact, the flu is about six times more likely to send you to the hospital if you have diabetes. This is why getting a flu shot before the winter flu season is so important for those with diabetes. Bronchitis and pneumonia are two potential complications of the flu that can be very dangerous. Your doctor may recommend a pneumonia vaccine every five or six years, especially for older folks with diabetes.

A Cold A stuffy nose, sneezing, and a sore throat are common signs of a cold. As with any illness, a cold can make your blood sugar rise, so it's important to test your sugar more often when you are sick.

An Infection You probably know that people with diabetes are at higher risk for all sorts of infections. A sinus infection, for example, can make your blood sugar rise, and high blood sugar can make an infection difficult to shake. If you take insulin, you might need to take an increased dose when you have an infection. Talk with your doctor to see if any adjustment is necessary.

Testing when ill
looking out for ketones

It's important to keep an eye out for low blood sugar (hypoglycemia) when you cannot keep food down, and the high blood sugar (hyperglycemia) that results from illness or injury. Most health care professionals recommend that you check blood sugar every two to four hours and keep a log of the results over the day. This log will be helpful when you speak with your doctor.

When you are sick, it's important to be on the lookout for ketones, by-products of your body's burning fat for energy. If your sugar gets very high, or when there's not enough food in your body for energy, ketones can build up in your bloodstream and spill into the urine. This can be very dangerous. If your blood sugar is over 250 mg/dl, you should check for ketones in your urine. You want to avoid **diabetic ketoacidosis** (or DKA), a medical emergency that occurs when you are dehydrated and the level of ketones in the blood is very high. DKA happens primarily with type 1 diabetes, but it can happen if you have type 2 diabetes. If you have moderate to large amounts of ketones when you test, it's time to call your doctor.

For a long time, the only way you could test for ketones at home was to dip specially treated plastic ketone testing strips, called ketostix, into some urine you had collected. This is not difficult, but it's kind of a drag to deal with; it's still the most common way to check for ketones.

A new method of checking for ketones allows you to use a blood sample instead of urine. And while that doesn't sound like the world's greatest trade-off, it's certainly a less awkward way to make sure your ketone level isn't too high and to keep yourself out of the hospital with ketoacidosis. Some advanced new blood-meters can check both blood sugar and ketones in the blood. You use one strip for your usual glucose testing and another kind of strip (in the same meter) for testing for blood ketones.

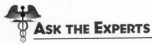

ASK THE EXPERTS

Why is my blood sugar so high? I haven't even eaten anything!

Any kind of stress, illness, or injury can make your body pour more glucose into your bloodstream. Hormones produced during illness can also cause blood sugar to rise. These spikes happen, but they are not your fault. And there's not much you can do about it except test your blood sugar more often when you are feeling sick. That's why it's really important to take your medicine, even when you cannot eat.

Don't stress out if your blood sugar is high. You are probably going to see some blood sugar readings that are hard to understand when you are not 100 percent. The best you can do is drink lots of water, test often, and check for ketones when your blood sugar is above 240 mg/dl. Work with your doctor to adjust your medicine on a sick day to try to avoid high blood sugar.

Can over-the-counter cold or flu medicines react with my diabetes?

Medicines you take for cold and flu symptoms, as well as those you take for infections, can affect blood sugar. Some antibiotics can lower blood sugar. And some decongestants can raise blood sugar. Ask your doctor or pharmacist to recommend a medicine for your symptoms, and find out whether it has an effect on your glucose levels so that you can compensate or find a suitable substitution. Sugar-free cough drops and liquid cough syrups are readily available now.

Over-the-counter medications
watch the sugar content

If you take insulin, you often need to increase your dose when you are sick to counter the extra glucose your body is putting into your bloodstream. So it's important to stick to your usual plan for taking insulin or diabetes pills, try to get about the same number of calories you normally do, and work with your doctor to make adjustments if necessary.

There are times when you may need to take less insulin, especially if you cannot eat and your blood sugar is running below 150 mg/dl. Frequent testing will help your doctor judge how your illness is affecting your diabetes and whether your medication should be adjusted.

When you walk into a pharmacy to find some sort of relief from your symptoms, it's often confusing to figure out what you can or cannot take. Ask the pharmacist about the sugar content of any over-the-counter medicines. Some, such as those that contain pseudoephedrine, may cause your blood sugar and blood pressure to rise, and should be avoided. Ask your doctor if you are concerned about side effects, and see if he or she can point out medicines that do not contain sugar. A number of over-the-counter medicines are available in sugar-free versions if you prefer not to have the excess sugar. Your pharmacist can also help you find sugar-free medicines or determine how an over-the-counter medicine you like to use might affect your blood sugar. If you check your sugar often, you should be able to compensate for the amount of sugar in cold and cough medicines. So if there's a medicine you particularly like that has sugar in it, you can probably still take it. Just check with your doctor.

Because illness can be especially hard on those with diabetes, it's a great idea to get a flu shot every year. The flu shot is effective, and it won't give you the flu. The American Diabetes Association recommends scheduling a flu shot in early September. Note that those who are allergic to eggs should not get a flu shot.

Common sugar-free medicines

◆ Cough Drops: Robitussin, Nice, Halls, Diabetic Tussin, Ricola, and Fisherman's Friend sugar-free cough drops or lozenges

◆ Cough Medicine: Diabetic Tussin DM, Robitussin Sugar-Free Cough Suppressant

◆ Allergies: Diabetic Tussin AL Allergy Relief

◆ Colds: Cold-Eeze Sugar Free Cold Medication

◆ Sore Throat: Chloraseptic Throat Spray

You will also commonly find inexpensive sugar-free store-brand cough drops.

FIRST PERSON INSIGHTS

Even brides get the flu

I was dizzy with details before my wedding. Between calling the caterer and the DJ, making arrangements for out-of-town guests, and worrying about how our families would get along, I forgot to get a flu shot. After the stress of planning, and late nights with friends and family, I was wiped out. A nasty bug was going around at the wedding, and, sure enough, two days after the big day, I got it. The problem was, I was in London, far from my doctor and my pharmacist. For two weeks during my honeymoon, I hobbled around England looking for medicines that were sugar-free and comparable to what I take at home. I'm still not sure what the product "Night Nurse" is supposed to do, but I took half a pack over my trip. I never shook the flu. Now I always get a yearly flu shot, and I absolutely won't travel until I've had it.

—Sara T., Akron, OH

Working from home
reducing stress means fewer sick days

In this modern world of faxes, cell phones, and e-mail, many people can at least occasionally work from home. When you are sick, the ability to work from home can be a real blessing. And telecommuting can relieve stress, which can help bring blood sugar levels into control overall. That's good news when illness or an injury is making your body kick up glucose production.

If you have a job that you can do from home, why wait until you get sick to set up a telecommuting arrangement with your boss? During your next employee evaluation or some other convenient time, explain to your employer that your diabetes could benefit from a work-at-home arrangement. If you are concerned that your boss will reject the idea, make sure to explain how you can meet all the requirements of your job from home. If you can reduce stress during the week, you are less likely to fall ill and miss days at work.

If you are worried your employer will react negatively to a telecommuting request, start small. Ask to telecommute one or two days out of the week. You might even find that you get more done in a relaxed atmosphere, on your own computer, when there are fewer distractions.

What about working with files? Ask an office friend to fax you materials that are only on paper. Or arrange your week so that you do e-mail and Internet-based work primarily on your day at home. Be creative. Don't let details hold you back if working from home is important to you.

Telecommuting Checklist

You may not have your home office set up yet, but you can create a good work space fairly easily. Here's what you will need.

◆ **An Internet connection.** If your office is using e-mail and the Web, you should be able to stay in touch with your employer and clients using e-mail software, such as Outlook Express or Eudora, which come free with your computer.

◆ **Remote-access software.** Programs including Traveling Software's LapLink (www.laplink.com) can help you copy files from home or office computer. Another option is a Web service called GoToMyPC (www.gotomypc.com), which allows you to access your computer at work from any computer that has Internet access and a Web browser. This is very handy when you are feeling under par but want to stay on top of things at headquarters.

◆ **A fax machine or fax software.** Newer computers often include fax software free with the operating system (as Windows XP does).

◆ **Database software** for maintaining contacts.

Going to the hospital
staying on track through a bad bout

M any people with diabetes worry that if they have to go to the hospital for some non–diabetes-related problem, the hospital staff won't provide diabetic medicine or diabetic meals in a timely way. If you have to stay in the hospital, remember that your normal diabetes regimen can, and likely will, be disrupted. The health care team there will provide your meals, test your blood sugar, and give you fast-acting glucose if you need it. That can be a little unnerving when you are used to running the show. Of course, you can still check your own blood sugar. Many patients on oral medication may be put on insulin while in the hospital. This does not mean they will be on insulin when they are discharged.

Along with your meter, here are a few other things to bring along if you need to go to the hospital:

- ◆ Fast-acting sugar or glucose tablets. If you prefer, take glucose gel (available at any pharmacy), which doesn't need to be chewed.

- ◆ Your glucose testing kit and supplies.

- ◆ Warm socks and slippers.

- ◆ Your insulin and/or diabetes pills. Note: Most hospitals will insist on using their own medications from a central pharmacy so they can monitor what you are getting.

- ◆ Your MedicAlert bracelet.

- ◆ Ketostix for testing ketones.

Sick-day checklist

◆ Stay in close contact with your doctor.

◆ Drink lots of liquids, about six to eight ounces an hour, to avoid dehydration.

◆ Avoid caffeine, and stick with herbal tea, water, or caffeine- and sugar-free soda. Be careful of beverages that are high in sugar, such as juice, which can drive your blood sugar higher.

◆ Check your sugar often (every two to four hours), and keep a log of the results.

◆ Expect changes in your eating habits. You may eat less while hospitalized. And, therefore, you may need to have your diabetes medications altered.

◆ Don't stop taking your medicine.

◆ Check for ketones if your blood sugar is over 240.

◆ Call your doctor if your blood sugar is over 240 twice in a row when you test or if you have ketones when you test.

◆ If you suffer vomiting or diarrhea, call your doctor.

◆ Don't exercise. Give your body a rest.

Helpful resources

American Diabetes Association
Complete Guide to Diabetes
Excellent information on sick-day
management from the folks at the
ADA. This small paperback is inexpensive (less than $7) and offers
wide-ranging coverage of diabetes
care.

ADA Recommendations:
Sick Day Type 2
www.diabetes.org/main/type2/liv
ing/sick/default.jsp

Preventing Complications

Knowing the risks
how to cut down on complications

The idea of diabetes-related complications is something you probably would rather avoid considering. Complications are scary and unpredictable. And while controlling your blood sugar and blood pressure is the best way to avoid and prevent complications, there's a wild card in the deck—it's still not clear why some people with diabetes are more prone to certain complications than others.

Short-term diabetic complications include hypoglycemia (low blood sugar) and hyperglycemia (high blood sugar). Low and high blood sugar are typically infrequent annoyances, but left untreated they can be life threatening. Uncontrolled diabetes, in which hyperglycemia is more often the norm than the exception, can lead to more serious problems.

Diabetic complications fall into two camps. First there are the macrovascular complications. These are diseases involving the larger blood vessels that, when left untreated, can kill. They are:

◆ **Heart disease**
◆ **Stroke**

Then there are those complications that involve the tiny blood vessels that link the arteries and veins; these are called microvascular complications. Left untreated, they can cause permanent disability. They are:

◆ **Nerve damage** (neuropathy)
◆ **Eye disease** (retinopathy)
◆ **Kidney disease** (nephropathy)

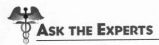

ASK THE EXPERTS

Why do people get complications?

Chronic high blood sugar is hard on the body. Hyperglycemia can restrict blood flow to the heart, increasing the risk of a heart attack, and to the brain, which can cause a stroke. It can wear out your kidneys and affect your vision. Often it's not completely clear why extra glucose in the blood harms various parts of your body, but the risk of diabetic complications resulting from long-term hyperglycemia is apparent in numerous studies.

How can I tell if a symptom I have is caused by diabetes or some other condition?

It's understandable that you might assume diabetes is the cause of most of your occasional ills. See a doctor immediately if you are concerned that you have a diabetic complication. But don't worry that every pain is diabetes related. Keep in mind that some complications are short term, and disappear when blood sugar is brought under control. Complications are much more successfully treated when caught early, so make sure to see your primary care physician and specialist on a regular basis, and try not to worry too much.

I really hate having to worry so much about my health. Isn't there a time for a bit of healthy denial?

Denial is a normal human response to tough situations, but it can lead to problems. In the case of diabetes, it can mean a delay in treating complications. Better to know what there is to worry about so you can begin to cope. Sure, at times you may feel overwhelmed, but there is power in knowing what you are up against.

Heart disease and stroke
why those with diabetes have a higher risk

Yes, diabetes plays havoc on the body's blood sugar. But who knew that the result of those blood sugar woes leads to a considerably increased risk of heart disease, heart attack, and stroke. In fact, whenever cardiologists see a patient with diabetes, they often treat him as if he had already a heart attack! For that reason, blood-pressure goals and cholesterol goals are lower for people with diabetes than for the general population. That translates into having blood pressure at less than 130/85 and LDL cholesterol levels at under 100. Control of blood pressure and cholesterol are as crucial to diabetes as controlling blood sugar.

Cardiovascular disease sometimes gets less attention than other diabetic complications. Yet, according to the American Diabetes Association, two out of three people with diabetes die from heart disease and stroke. That's an alarming figure, but there are ways to greatly improve the odds.

As you age, your risk increases. The risk is even greater if you smoke or have high blood pressure or a high cholesterol count. The combination of obesity and an inactive lifestyle also spells trouble.

So, how can you reduce your risk of heart disease and stroke? Eating a healthy diet and losing weight are good places to start. It's important to watch the fat and cholesterol in meat and dairy products and to eat a high-fiber diet. And the risk of heart disease and stroke is yet another good reason not to smoke. Quitting smoking will reduce blood pressure and improve cholesterol. Finally, controlling your diabetes can help prevent or delay the damage to your blood vessels that high blood sugar can cause.

Let's look on the bright side: It's not all bad news here. An aspirin a day (check with your doctor first) can help by thinning your blood and helping to reduce blood clots. Also, studies show that a glass of wine a day can increase your good-cholesterol (or HDL) level.

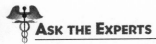

ASK THE EXPERTS

I heard that some people with diabetes don't have the same warning signs of a heart attack as everyone else. Is that true?

There are conflicting reports on this matter. Some studies suggest that, many people are unable to correctly identify chest pain that is a warning sign of a heart attack, whether they have diabetes or not. This is a disturbing thought—that people might be unaware of this symptom and fail to rush to an emergency room. If you feel pain or tightness in your chest, or pain that runs from your chest into your jaw, left arm, or shoulder, chew an aspirin (if you are not allergic) and call an ambulance immediately. Some people with diabetes who have had a heart attack report feeling sick to their stomach or short of breath—even when they didn't feel chest pain. Remember: You have to act fast to protect your heart.

Are there signs that I may be headed for a heart attack or stroke?

You have diabetes, and you know that's a risk factor. If you find that your cholesterol, A_{1c}, and blood pressure are higher than normal, you need to act quickly to get back on track. People with diabetes are more likely to suffer heart attacks and strokes, and these occur earlier in life. When these three tests are out of whack, you could be headed for trouble. If this is the case, talk to your physician about changing your treatment plan.

Neuropathy
fending off nerve damage

It's not completely clear why people with diabetes sometimes develop nerve damage. As with other complications, long-term hyperglycemia increases the risk. Over time, too much glucose in the blood can damage the cells that cover the nerves and damage blood vessels, reducing the oxygen brought to the nerves.

You can help prevent nerve damage with good blood sugar control. The Diabetes Control and Complications Trial (DCCT), a study of 1,441 individuals from 1983 to 1989, showed that the risk of neuropathy could be reduced by 60 percent through tighter blood sugar control. If you already have some damage, better blood glucose control can help prevent further damage and even help reverse some symptoms of neuropathy.

Sensory Neuropathy Hyperglycemia over time can cause pain or numbness in nerves, usually in the arms, legs, and hands. After a while, the tingling or burning sensation can give way to loss of sensation, which makes it more likely that an injury to the area will go unnoticed.

Autonomic Neuropathy is damage to the nerves that regulate such body functions as blood flow, digestion, and heart rate. This form of nerve damage can cause difficulty in areas of your body that you don't control, including digestion, urination, blood pressure, and sexual function.

It's important to check your feet every day for cuts or sores. If you have a cut or sore that doesn't heal in two or three days, you should seek medical attention. If you have nerve damage, infections take much longer to heal, and this can can have serious consequences—namely, amputation.

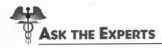

ASK THE EXPERTS

How can I tell if I've got neuropathy?

Your doctor can perform a neurological evaluation when you get your checkup. One of the first signs of neuropathy is loss of sensation, which can be tested using a tuning fork to see if you can sense vibration. Your doctor may check your ankle reflexes, as well as prick your feet to test sensation.

Can neuropathy affect my sex life? Tell me the answer is no.

There is good news and bad news. Neuropathy can cause vaginal dryness, which can be helped with lubricants. Neuropathy can also cause impotence in men. Discuss with your doctor the possibility of prescribing a drug that will enable an erection when taken before sex enhance libido in women.

FIRST PERSON INSIGHTS

Better to speak up

I noticed a painful tingling sensation in my feet sometimes during a period of my life when I was under a lot of stress and my blood glucose levels were often very high. The sensation went away when my blood sugar came down. I was scared to even mention this to my doctor, but I did. He explained that there is an acute form of neuropathy that can be controlled by getting blood glucose levels back to normal. Doing so can also help reduce the risk of pain and muscle weakness caused by long-term nerve damage, and this brush with neuropathy has been a major reason I watch my blood sugar more carefully now that my life has settled down a bit.

—Terry W., Portland, ME

Retinopathy
caring for your eyes

If your doctor says that you have signs of retinopathy, you can take heart that you are not alone. About 90 percent of people with diabetes have some form of blood-vessel change in their eyes after having diabetes for 25 years. The first signs of retinopathy do not mean you are headed for imminent vision loss. Good glucose control, early detection, and modern treatments—if necessary—have a huge impact on maintaining good vision.

Simply put, hyperglycemia over a long period of time, along with high blood pressure, can cause damage to your retina, the lining in the back of the eye that senses light. Tiny blood vessels in the retina can break and leak blood into the fluid in the back of the eye.

There are two types of retinopathy:

Nonproliferative retinopathy is a relatively common condition among people who have had diabetes for many years. In this form of retinopathy, capillaries expand and form pouches that are visible during an eye exam. It does not require treatment.

Proliferative retinopathy can result when blood vessels are damaged by chronic hyperglycemia. This more serious condition can cause new blood vessels to grow in order to carry the blood. But these new blood vessels are weak and may leak blood into the eye, clouding your vision. Without treatment, this can lead to blindness.

Diabetes is also linked to a greater risk of **glaucoma,** where pressure increases on the optic nerve, and **cataracts,** clouding of the eye. Both conditions are treatable but need to be caught early to fight off vision loss. These are two more good reasons to see your ophthalmologist. And if you experience problems, know that there are effective treatments.

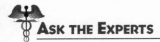

ASK THE EXPERTS

How often should I be checked for retinopathy?

Your ophthalmologist should dilate your eyes and check the back of your eyes once a year, and more often if you have signs of retinopathy. Your primary care physician should check your eyes each time you meet, but you still need to see an eye-care specialist yearly.

How can I prevent retinopathy?

You probably know that keeping your blood sugar as close to normal as possible will help. It's also important to watch your blood pressure, as high blood pressure increases the risk of getting eye disease.

What should I do if I have retinopathy?

As you might expect, your health team will likely encourage you to tighten your blood glucose control, which can help. Outpatient laser surgery to seal blood vessels is routinely used and may dramatically reduce the risk of blindness.

Nephropathy
avoiding kidney disease

Your kidneys are extremely capable of filtering toxins from your blood. In fact, they are so good, kidney disease can be present for many years before any symptoms occur. They will continue to function despite poorly controlled diabetes and high blood pressure, although damage will ensue. If your blood pressure and/or blood glucose remain chronically too high, the kidneys cannot properly filter toxins from your blood. The blood vessels leak protein into the urine instead of returning it to the blood. The result is kidney disease. In end-stage kidney disease, when the kidneys have lost most of their ability to function, dialysis is typically recommended. There are two types of dialysis:

Hemodialysis removes blood from an artery, detoxifies it in a machine, and returns it through a vein. The process typically requires a short surgical procedure to insert a device called a shunt into the artery. The procedure typically takes two to four hours, several times a week. Dialysis takes place at a hospital or a dialysis facility.

In **peritoneal dialysis**, a fluid is inserted through a tube into the abdominal cavity, where the fluid, called **dialysate**, collects toxins. The fluid is then drained out through the tube. Peritoneal dialysis can be done at home, often overnight while you sleep.

Another, perhaps more attractive and effective, option is a kidney transplant, often from a family member. In the case of a patient with diabetes and kidney failure, a simultaneous kidney and pancreas transplant is recommended. This type of transplant essentially cures the diabetes, which will increase the success of the kidney transplant. The catch is that transplant recipients must take antirejection drugs every day for the rest of their lives to fight off rejection of their new organs, which their body treats as foreign objects.

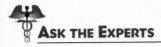

ASK THE EXPERTS

How often should I be tested for signs of kidney disease?

There are blood tests your doctor can use to check your kidney function. Your doctor should test for protein in the urine once a year.

What do I do if I have kidney disease?

Maintaining good glucose control and keeping blood pressure normal will help. A low-protein diet, developed by your doctor or dietitian, can help slow the progression of kidney disease. If you have high blood pressure or signs of protein in your urine, your doctor may prescribe medicine to lower your blood pressure, which can delay the progress of kidney disease. Your doctor may also recommend that you reduce your salt intake and will likely recommend that you exercise daily or several times a week.

Helpful resources

Thyroid Foundation of America, Inc.
Tel: 800 832-8321
Fax: 617 534-1515
www.allthyroid.org

American Foundation of Thyroid Patients
Tel: 432 694-9966
www.thyroidfoundation.org

Merck Manual of Medical Information
www.merck.com

Gland Central
(Internet source of thyroid information)
glandcentral.com

The American Diabetes Association
A nonprofit organization that promotes education, advocacy, and research. The ADA's *Diabetes Forecast* is a monthly magazine that offers tips for management and articles on research.
www.diabetes.org

The Insulin-Free World Foundation is a cure-focused organization that promotes research on islet and pancreas transplants and works to create a community of diabetics who have received, or want more information about, transplants. The IFW's Web site also offers handy information on insulin-pump therapy.
www.insulinfree.org

The Juvenile Diabetes Research Foundation
A nonprofit organization like the ADA, the JDRF provides information and advice for people with type 1 diabetes. The organization raises money, funds research, and lobbies for legislation that benefits people with diabetes. Mary Tyler Moore (diagnosed with type 1 at age 30) has long been the JDRF's chairperson. The JDRF puts out a monthly magazine, *Countdown,* that accompanies membership.
www.jdrf.org

On *Stress* and *Comfort*

What is stress?
it's not just a built-in survival mechanism

The alarm rings. You wake up startled and head for the shower. Then it's coffee and the morning rush. On and on it goes, until you come home staggering and exhausted. Welcome to the world of chronic stress. Not surprisingly, *stress* has become the watchword of the millennium.

Now stress researchers are learning that stress can cause certain illnesses as well as worsen your symptoms once you become ill. How can stress cause illness as well as worsen its symptoms? The answer lies in the very complex nature of stress—or, rather, our complex reaction to it. While scientists have learned a great deal more about the nature of stress in the past few years, they are still baffled by it. One of the most puzzling aspects of stress is that its effect on our bodies is based on how we perceive stressful situations. Some stress can help us perform at our peak abilities, such as competing in a race, while other stress can be debilitating, such as an unwanted divorce or a job loss. It's all in the eye of the beholder.

A perceived short-term threat

When it comes to short-term stress, there is a fairly universal understanding of it. In fact, surviving a sudden threat is so critical to our survival that our bodies are designed to either fight or flee the threat. This short-term stressor could be a lunging tiger, an oncoming car, or an angry boss. Here's how our bodies handle it: When a threat is perceived, the brain's hypothalamus sends out an alarm to the sympathetic nervous system to release adrenaline into the bloodstream. This increases your heart rate and blood pressure so you can run or fight. It also drains blood from the brain. That means the brain is getting less oxygen, and this in turn makes rational thinking a lot harder. (Ever wonder why people sometimes freeze in the face of danger or do something really irrational? It's because they get so light-headed they literally cannot think of what to do.)

Next, the brain signals the adrenal glands to release epinephrine and norepinephrine hormones. These hormones increase the glucose levels in the blood so that muscles can effectively respond. This is why some people perform incredible feats of strength in a crisis. Note: The perceived threat is always in the eye of the beholder. The stress response will occur whether the threat is real or imagined. (This is why your heart races during a scary movie.)

Once the threat has passed, the brain issues an "all-clear" signal. Neurons, special cells in the brain, send out signals to the major organs to return to normal. This allows the digestive system to go back to the business of digesting food, and the heart's rate and your blood pressure are told to return to a calmer beat. Essentially, the body is told to relax—the threat has passed. If the threat lasted for a few minutes, it will take just a few minutes to return to normal.

Women and Stress

Women react differently to stress

For the past 50 years, stress research was done on male animals. It was from their response to various stressors that researchers came up with the catch phrase fight or flight. That changed in 1998, when researcher Shelley E. Taylor thought to study the stress response in female animals. Dr. Taylor found that females responded differently to non–life-threatening stress, particularly if they were tending young offspring. These animals did not become nearly as alarmed as their male counterparts. In fact, their reaction was to tend to their young and to seek comfort in other females. Dr. Taylor went on to test her theory on men and women and found that in general men tend to isolate themselves when they feel stressed, while women confide their problems to each other. As Dr. Taylor describes it in her book, The Tending Instinct, women "tend and befriend."

Chronic stress
be alert to coping patterns

What happens when a perceived threat lingers for days or weeks? Long-term negative stressors, such as a messy divorce, becoming ill, or being laid off from work, go on for months. This means the all-clear signal is never given by the brain, so the body never gets a chance to return to equilibrium. It's as if the body is in a constant state of alert. Over time, this can take a physical toll on the body, especially if these stressors are perceived to be negative threats. Again, perception is key. This is why some people thrive on such stressors as deadlines for a project they are passionate about, and why others who don't feel emotionally involved or in control of their work feel "stressed out."

When it comes to long-term stress, having a sense of control is key. Long-term negative stress can lead to bouts of anxiety, aggression, and depression. Some scientists believe that chronic stress has a harmful effect on the immune system and the endocrine system, making people more vul-nerable to illness and infections. Having an illness can be very stressful. People with diabetes tend to have more anxiety and cases of depression than the general population. Does this mean they are more sensitive to the effects of stress? Most likely, yes.

How do you cope with the chronic stress of having a chronic illness? For starters, look at how you have coped in the past with other chronic stres-sors, especially negative ones. Did you isolate yourself from friends and family? Did you seek out comfort foods? sleep a lot? fall into bad habits, such as overeating or drinking? Try to see if there is a pattern to how you coped. It's also a good idea to recall how your parents or other significant caregivers handled negative stressors. You may have internalized their cop-ing responses and not realized it.

Negative Coping Responses

There are several negative coping responses that we all have used at one time or another when dealing with long-term stress. Here's a roundup:

◆ **Deny the problem.** This is a common response for many people—they simply ignore the problem. Often, to help take their minds off the problem, they throw themselves into their work or social life.

◆ **Dwell on your problems.** Again, this is usually a learned response. Did your parents or caregivers fret excessively over your health as you were growing up? Or did they ignore your health completely? If they did either of these extremes, you may find yourself obsessing about your health. If these thoughts become chronic, you should see a therapist who can help you break the pattern of obsessive rumination.

◆ **Procrastinate decision making.** Instead of thinking through the problems at hand, you endlessly analyze the situations and talk about the same problems and solutions over and over again with friends and family.

◆ **Seek thrills.** Here you look for excitement or experiences to distract you from your problems.

◆ **Get angry and vent to others.** This is known as displaced aggression. It's when you take out your anger at being ill on others and overreact to their responses.

◆ **Withdraw.** Physically or emotionally withdraw from others. Often people under chronic stress will cope by sleeping excessively or simply by disengaging from the world.

◆ **Overindulge. Overeat.** Here food is used as a drug to mask fears as well as boredom. Too much alcohol is another way to cope with all the problems of a chronic illness.

Smart coping strategies
find positive ways to cope with chronic problems

Having a chronic illness can tap your coping reserves. Your old favorite coping standbys may work, but not for the long haul. The challenge of coping with long-term stress is understanding how to live with it. This calls for a new way of looking at your health and looking at illness. Since there is no cure as yet for many of the chronic illnesses we are heir to, the goal becomes the reduction of your discomfort. That means really listening to your symptoms and addressing them. Your goal is simply to improve your quality of life. Here are some coping tips to help you on your way:

Focus on favorite activities. If certain hobbies or activities, such as cooking a gourmet meal, going to the movies, playing sports, or reading mystery stories, were your means of getting away from it all in the past, chances are they will still do the trick. Moreover, they now can be a retreat from your new stress.

Get organized. Time management becomes a tool you can really use when you have a chronic illness. Your time and energy are now precious commodities that should not be wasted. Learn how to separate out those things you really need to do from those you can spread out over time or delegate to others.

Develop healthy habits. Ironically, people often become healthier once they have been diagnosed with a chronic illness. This may be because they suddenly stop taking their health for granted and turn negative habits into healthy ones, such as maintaining a good diet (see pages 83–104) or quitting smoking.

Make attitude adjustments. Life with chronic stress can make the world a dour place. Put some humor back in your life. Rent funny movies and read humorous books and magazines.

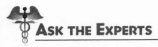

I have to travel for my work. How can I cut down on stress while I am on the road?

Traveling is a big stressor, doubly so if you have to manage a chronic illness while you are on the road. It's smart to be proactive and plan ahead as much as possible. For starters, always try to bring a few clothes and items from home that spell comfort to you. This could be a pair of old jeans or a favorite shawl. Some people who hate to travel take a lot of comfort in putting photographs of their family in their hotel room.

While in the plane, car, bus, or train, have a carry-on bag that has a favorite sweater, a CD player with headphones, an eye mask, a bottle of water, and some healthy snacks. Also create a mini-folder in which to store the phone numbers and contact information of all the people on your support team (see pages 67–82). Keep this folder with you at all times.

Can pets reduce stress?

There is some evidence that pets can reduce stress and hypertension. In one six-month study at the University of Buffalo, participants who adopted a dog or cat saw blood pressure caused by mental stress rise less than that of those who did not have a pet. Both the group with pets and the group without took an ACE inhibitor, a commonly prescribed means of controlling overall blood pressure. But when asked to take stress-inducing tests, such as giving a speech or doing arithmetic problems, the pet-owning group fared better when their blood pressure was taken.

Learning to relax
beat chronic stress at its own game

Our bodies are brilliantly designed to handle stress. They are also designed to handle relaxation. In fact, the stress response and the relaxation response are both hardwired into our brains. Doctors are just now beginning to understand the power of relaxation on the body—both to rejuvenate and to heal.

Think back to a time when you felt truly relaxed. What was going on? You were probably in a quiet, comfortable space where you had no pressure to do anything but to sit back and enjoy the day. You felt peaceful and at one with the world. For most people, that's the definition of a vacation. Here's the news flash: To be healthy, your body needs a little vacation every day. How do you achieve that? Here are some tips:

Develop quiet time. Carve out 10 minutes of the day to simply sit quietly and "be." Meditation practices are very helpful in teaching people how to quiet their minds and relax (see pages 110–115 for more on this).

Do some deep breathing. When you are stressed, your breathing becomes shortened, so much so that you can hyperventilate when faced with acute stress. Counter this natural instinct by purposefully taking four deep breaths every time you feel stressed. Breathe in through your nose, hold the breath for five seconds, and then release the air through your mouth.

Exercise. Chronic muscle tension is part and parcel of a chronic stress response. Counteract it by taking a walk or playing a round of tennis. Your goal is to keep your body limber and to keep it moving. For a more relaxing exercise, consider taking a class in yoga or tai chi (see pages 114–115 for more information). Note: Massage is a great way to help rid your muscles of stress-related tension (see pages 108–109).

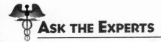

ASK THE EXPERTS

I have been anxious for so long, nothing helps. What can I do?

If you have been enduring chronic stressors for a long period of time, trying to relax overnight is not going to work. In fact, it will just make you more stressed. You need to retrain your body on how to feel and behave while relaxed. Consider taking a short-term workshop to help you learn how to relax. Your doctor can refer you to a stress-management clinic or a stress specialist. You might also take courses on stress management. The American Diabetes Management Association offers two-day workshops on managing stress—call them at 800-262-9699. Or try your local YMCA or YMHA; they usually offer stress-management classes.

I hear writing about stressful events helps you get over them. True?

There are some studies that show that writing about stressful issues or traumatic experiences can help improve the immune system. Use your health journal (see pages 22–23) to write about your concerns.

Talking about it
learn how to talk about your needs

For a lot of people, talking about their health issues is difficult. They don't want to come across as a whiner, nor do they want to seem overly dramatic. And so they say nothing. If this sounds familiar, then it's time to learn how to talk about having a chronic illness. If you don't learn how to talk about it, you risk isolating yourself from your friends, family, and coworkers, and cutting them out of a major part of your life. Your friends would feel left out if you didn't tell them that you got married or that one of your parents died. The same is true for a chronic illness. Not telling can erode your relationships, and the distance that can ensue will send you down the road to depression. Yes, it's hard to learn how to talk about having any problem, but you can do it. Here are a few tips to make it easier:

1. Pick the time and place to talk. You need to set a time and place that is comfortable for you. Don't get backed into talking about your illness when you are not ready. You need to feel in control of the conversation, and picking the place and time will help you feel in charge.

2. Rehearse out loud in front of a mirror before you actually talk to your family members or friends. Saying the words you want to say can help take the sting out of them. Call a diabetes center and find a counselor you can speak with.

3. Set the terms and limits of the information you want to share. You are the one in charge here; don't let anyone take over the conversation and ask you invasive questions. Simply call a halt to the questions and say you don't feel comfortable answering them right now. Also, set the terms of your information. If you don't want this information shared with others, then say so. Here's an example: "Joanie, I have been wanting to talk to you about something important that is going on in my life. At this time, I don't want this information shared with others. Is that okay with you?"

Learn how not to talk about it

It's only natural to assume that because something interests you intensely, then it must also interest everyone else. And if that something is as all-important as your health, your family and close friends will surely want to know every detail, and even casual acquaintances will be fascinated by the dramatic story line. Wrong. Remind yourself every day that a good conversationalist is first of all a good listener. Ask questions about things that interest other people, and listen—really listen—to the answers.

Six Rules for Talking About Your Illness

1. "How are you?" is a salutation, not a request for medical news. Just because you have a chronic illness, there's no reason to change your usual response. Wait until someone asks specifically about your illness before telling them about it.

2. Fit the answer to your audience. Have a short version and a long version ready. Your spouse may want to hear every detail the minute you come from your doctor's visit, but your colleagues want only a brief version.

3. Watch for eyes glazing over. Someone has asked about your illness and seems really interested. So you launch into the long version. Watch for signs that you may have misjudged. Does she fidget? Glance around? If you pause or ask a question, is there a slight delay before you have her attention again?

4. After three minutes, change the subject. Even the most loving friend may not be able to take in every detail of an extended medical report. Give her a break. If someone is really interested, she'll return to the subject.

5. Use humor. Have a couple of jokes handy to break up your monologue or provide an exit line.

6. Act interested. When someone tells you about their illness or operation, show interest. Remind yourself that it's your turn to be a listener. And try not to fidget.

Your partner's concerns
how chronic illness can impact relationships

Having an illness usually calls for couples to reassess their partnership. If it's a temporary illness, then it's usually a question of juggling practical matters, such as "Who will pick up the kids while I am at the doctor?" It's when symptoms are no longer the signs of a temporary illness but the manifestation of a chronic illness, that a bigger reassessment is needed. Couples need to look at each partner's role and responsibilities in the relationship. You need to state what changes you need to make. This may mean reassigning roles, whether cleaning duties or paying the bills. Often couples fall into the trap in which one becomes the dominant caregiver and the other becomes the professional patient. Try to avoid that dynamic because it usually leads to resentment on both sides. It's a good idea to have your spouse come along with you on a doctor visit in order to see firsthand what it is like to be a patient.

Money may become an issue if you don't have adequate health insurance or need to cut back on work (see pages 124–125). Chronic illness can also affect your sex lives. Long-term diabetes has been associated with impotence and reduced sexual sensation—but being diagnosed with diabetes is not a sentence of sexual dysfunction. Rather, it is one more reason to follow your daily regimen carefully and conscientiously. Talk about your concerns and listen to your partner. The important thing is to keep the lines of communication open, and not shut down. A good therapist, knowledgeable about the effects of chronic disease on sexuality, may be able to help you work through these issues. To find a therapist for your particular concern, start at the American Association of Sex Educators, Counselors, and Therapists (**www.aasect.org**). Also, check with the larger diabetes support foundations to see if they host any spouse-support groups. One resource is **www.diabetes.about.com**.

How to talk about your chronic illness

How do you tell your children that you have a chronic illness? It depends on how much this illness has impacted your health. In the case of diabetes, you need to tell your children in simple terms what diabetes is, how it affects you, and what you need to do to manage it.

If you have young children, pick a quiet time and place to talk about it. Ask your partner to be present at this meeting. Use easy-to-understand language. Be as specific as you can: "Remember when Mommy couldn't take you to the swimming pool because she was too tired? Well, the reason is that Mommy has an illness, but she is getting better. We need to work out together how to do some things. Let's ask Aunt Sandy or Uncle Mike to take you to the swimming pool. How does that sound?"

Older children will want to know more details. Again, be specific; use concrete examples of how the illness has affected you. Rehearse what you want to say. The most important thing is to assure your children that you are not in any danger. Reassure them that you and they will be just fine.

Managing the inconveniences
dealing with the hard issues

There are a number of inconveniences involved when you have a chronic illness. They usually come down to two things: time and money. If your symptoms are still troubling you, you are bound to find yourself canceling social engagements or perhaps rearranging your work schedule. Then, of course, there are the many doctor appointments you need to factor into your already busy schedule. This is not fun.

Next comes a real stressor for those with a chronic illness: paying for it. If you do not have health insurance, having a chronic illness can be very costly. You will need to find low-cost clinics to help you manage your illness. And since diabetes requires lifelong management, you will need to find low-cost sources of insulin and blood-sugar-testing supplies that you can afford. If you are over 65, you can apply for Medicare. For those with health insurance, the stress focuses on the myriad forms you will need to present to get coverage for your health care.

FIRST PERSON INSIGHTS

The power of a metaphor

I wanted to explain to my cousin what it was like to have type 1 diabetes. He could never understand why I avoided certain activities, like drinking with his buddies or crabbing barefoot. Finally one day, I hit upon a way to explain it to him. I knew he would understand what being laid off felt like. Well, I told him having a chronic illness is a lot like getting laid off. In both cases, it happens through "no fault of your own." And there is this sense of being an outsider—you miss your work routine and feel cut off from the "normal" working world. You are also concerned about your future and anxious to get back to work. I told him that is what having diabetes is like; sometimes it forces you out of regular everyday things. He got it. Ever since then, he's stopped hassling me about my choices.

—Chuck J., Chicago, IL

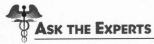

I am between jobs and don't have any health insurance right now. How do I find inexpensive health insurance that will cover my pre-existing diabetes?

You want to consider health-insurance coverage that is based on membership instead of employment. Consider joining a trade or professional organization that has its own health insurance. For example, if you are a graphic artist, you can join the AIGA, the American Institute of Graphic Artists. It has an insurance plan for its members, and once you join you can become eligible for it.

I have had to miss a couple of days to undergo tests. Should I tell my boss about my diabetes?

This is totally up to you. It is not necessary to go "public" about your health to your employer, unless your performance at work is suffering because of it. Only you can know that. Everyone gets sick from time to time. You should not be made to feel guilty about taking your allotted sick days. If you find you need more time off because of your diabetes, then, yes, you do need to explain your situation to your boss. Thanks to the Americans with Disabilities Act, once you inform your employer about your health condition, you cannot be fired because of it. You need to work with your boss to accommodate both your health needs and the needs of the business (see pages 138–139 for information about telecommuting).

Helpful resources

The Chronic Illness Workbook
by Patricia Fennel

The Tending Instinct
by Shelley E. Tayler

*Difficult Conversations: How to
Discuss What Matters Most*
by Douglas Stone, Sheila Heen, and
Bruce Patton

Stress and Diabetes
www.diabetes.about.com/cs/
stressdiabetes
About.com's helpful list of resources
for dealing with the day-to-day
stresses of living with diabetes.

The New You

Life with diabetes
it can be a rocky road

In your not too distant past, whenever you got sick, you went to the doctor, got a prescription, felt better, and went on with your life. That changed the day you got the diagnosis that you had diabetes. When you are first diagnosed, it's hard to see how you will adjust to the fundamental changes diabetes requires. There are days (especially when your blood sugar is out of whack) when you wonder when you will ever feel "normal" again. The reality is that for you, now, having diabetes is normal.

Like other major changes in your life, such as switching careers or becoming a parent, the adjustment to life as an individual with diabetes can be rough. But don't think you're alone. A quick Internet search of diabetes mailing lists and newsgroups (see pages 45–66) will show you just how common diabetes-inspired frustration can be. Don't let raging blood sugar make you think you cannot handle diabetes. You can, and you will.

Eventually, your emotions will stabilize as you begin to work diabetes into your everyday life. You will feel more in control when you are watching your diet, exercise, and blood sugar, and you realize you can manage your new life without freaking out over every misstep: a high blood sugar reading, for example, or an occasionally forgotten diabetes pill. Go easy on yourself, even when everyone is wagging a finger in your direction. You are in charge here. Things will calm down as you get the hang of your treatment.

Learning how to talk about changes in your symptoms is key. A lot of people have trouble with this (see pages 8–9). But ignoring your symptoms can be downright dangerous. There's a fine line between paying attention to your symptoms and dwelling on them. You may never return to your pre-diagnosis self, and that takes time to absorb. There are a lot of changes to keep track of. This is one reason your doctor will ask if your symptoms are interfering with your daily life. Keeping a health journal can help you track your feelings and symptoms (see pages 22–23).

Remember, your diagnosis and the changes that come with it throw some big changes at your family, too. Your better half can feel a little overwhelmed with all there is to learn. The way you shop, cook, and eat may be substantially different now. And, remember, your spouse is probably just as worried about your health and possible complications as you are. Perhaps even more so if he or she doesn't have all the information.

Also bear in mind that even though your illness has been diagnosed and is now under control, your health problems are not over. If nothing else, aging will exacerbate your symptoms, as can major life changes, such as having children, the death of loved ones, moving house. If you can accept diabetes as a lifelong challenge that you can embrace into your life, you are much more likely to prevent complications.

FIRST PERSON INSIGHTS

It's not just your disease

A few months after I was first diagnosed with type 1, my wife and I were awakened by a doozy of a rainstorm, but I didn't know it at the time. I remember seeing erratic flashes of light bouncing off our bedroom walls and this super loud crashing all around. My heart started racing, and my palms felt sweaty. When it happened again, I turned to my wife. "What do you think that was?" I asked nervously. "Um, thunder," she said sleepily. Then she reached over to the nightstand and handed me my little glucose meter. "Why don't you check your blood sugar?" she suggested. I did. It was at 52, about half what it should have been. As I headed to the kitchen for a glass of juice to correct my low, I caught a glimpse of my reflection in the toaster chrome. My hair was sticking up everywhere. My eyes looked big as saucers. Little beads of sweat clung to my forehead. I guess my wife was getting used to my diabetes, learning the symptoms of low blood sugar better than I was. I appreciate that she can help me figure out what's normal when I don't feel normal.

—Gene W., Park City, UT

Stages of adjustment
from the old you to the new you

Attitude is everything. As doctors start to realize the healing power of the mind, they are paying more attention to helping their patients better cope with chronic illness. Accepting that you have a medical condition is the first step. This is not as easy as it sounds. Some researchers believe that coping with a chronic illness entails grieving over one's lost health. There is a range of emotions to go through, and they are similar to those explained by Elisabeth Kübler Ross in her groundbreaking book *On Death and Dying*. Those stages of grief are anger, denial, bargaining, depression, and acceptance. There is no prescribed order or set time to these stages.

Denial

Once you get that diagnosis, you realize that your illness is something you will always need to be aware of. You can no longer take your health for granted, even though diabetes is treatable. This is a bitter pill for some people to swallow, especially young people who have never had a health issue. Not surprisingly, they often choose to ignore it. Some go so far as not to take their medication. Or they eat too much. Or throw themselves into work instead of watching their diet and blood sugar. What's the reason for this? For most people it's fear. The symptoms of diabetes can be very frightening. There's a loss of personal power, which is an important contributor to self-esteem. There's also a loss of independence because managing your diabetes may interfere with how you normally live your life. Going back to your doctor for a new treatment plan seems futile, or so you think. You opt to deny any problems. Don't.

What to do: Be kind to yourself. Coping with all these issues can be overwhelming. Every person who has experienced strange medical symptoms is very frightened. What would you tell a friend who was experiencing strange physical symptoms? Probably the same thing your family and friends are telling you. Something is wrong. Seek help. See your doctor.

Anger, Depression, and Bargaining

You're mad at everything and everyone. "I see my doctors for my diabetes checkups. I do everything they tell me to do. And I still don't feel good. This just isn't fair!" Plus, your friends and family go on as if your problem doesn't exist, and that makes you mad. After all, it's not as if you have a "capital-S" serious illness. You're not going to die from this thing. But no one seems to understand how upset you feel. You cry and feel sorry for yourself and find no joy in any activity. Sorrow can lead to depression and destructive feelings. Chances are, you try to bargain your way out of this problem. "If I become a vegetarian, I will be healthy again. If I lose the weight I gained, everything will go back to the way it was." Bargaining is a favorite tool of just about everybody—not only those dealing with a chronic illness. The problem with bargaining is that it doesn't work; it's just another name for magical thinking.

What to do: The hard truth about coping with any chronic problem is that it is always there. The good news is that you will have some great days. And, conversely, you will have some not-so-great days, depending on how you respond to treatment. Being angry about that is normal—in fact, it's healthy. It's also okay to be sad and depressed. You didn't ask for this health problem, and it's okay to take some time for a little self-pity (see pages 160–161 for coping strategies that can ease you through the rough days). If you find that you are dwelling on your health more than you want to, consider seeing a therapist who can help you through these stages of adjustment (see page 77).

Acceptance
it doesn't happen in a day

Learning to accept a chronic disorder as part of your life is not easy. You miss the old carefree you. You miss not having to think about your health. You now fully understand why your grandparents used to say, "Don't take your health for granted." And you know what you have to do. With that knowledge comes a certain amount of power. It gives you back control over your life. Yes, you have this disorder, but it's treatable and it need not define who you are. You are still you, just a bit different thanks to your diabetes. And it's a different life than the one you had originally planned before you got this problem, but that's okay. The point is to work with this new reality and make it your own. Your job now is to recraft your life. How do you do this? It's not easy. It calls for a great deal of self-exploration. Think of it as a personal journey. Social workers and therapists who have counseled people with chronic illnesses suggest the following:

Learn about your condition

For some people, becoming a student of their condition can be an important way to get a sense of control back. They feel empowered learning the new vocabulary and finding out the latest news on the Internet. But for others, reading up on their illness or surfing the Internet can be very stressful. Still others go on a research binge, searching out everything available about diabetes treatments. If you're consumed by finding a cure for diabetes, it can be disheartening. Find your happy knowledge medium.

Get your support team together

In the beginning, it's important to find the right doctors and other support (see pages 67–82). These are the people who will be helping you regain your life. You need to find doctors who will partner with you in your long-term care. Sometimes the chemistry is not there. Keep looking until you find the right doctors who can communicate effectively with you.

Try to define what you have lost and gained

Think about the pattern of your symptoms. Have they kept you from doing things you would like to do? Make a list of those things. Now think about what not doing those things means to you. Are there any alternative ways to regain, or achieve, some of what you have lost? For a lot of people with diabetes, fatigue and drowsiness are the big hurdles. Feeling tired can impact your exercise routine, your dating life, your work life. You need to look at how things have changed since you were diagnosed before you can make new plans. As the authors of *Recrafting Your Life* explain it, you need to "figure out which parts of [your] old life you *can* continue and which you *want* to continue."

Avoid energy-draining situations

Keeping up your energy level is vital to maintaining a sense of purpose throughout your day. Don't let anything drain it unnecessarily. Sift through your typical day. Are there any particular times or places or people that make you uncomfortable? Try to identify them and see what you can do to turn things around. For example, if you find driving to work tires you out, consider other means of transport, such as carpooling, in which you don't have to do the driving all the time. If you notice your fatigue is at its highest at the end of the day, then plan on taking a rest then. Tell your family or roommates that you need a half hour of downtime and that you should not be disturbed.

Seek spiritual renewal

Having a chronic health condition can also make you cherish life more because you have learned not to take it for granted. For many this is the first time they have ever questioned the meaning of their life. To that end, seek out books, poems, plays, and movies about people who have overcome great odds. These heroic stories can do wonders for your spirit.

Overcoming setbacks
bumps along the way

Diabetes can feel like a never-ending series of speed bumps. Between blood glucose testing, dieting, enforced exercise, and the moodiness that comes with blood sugar highs and lows, diabetes seems constantly to interfere with your life. Sickness seems to hit you harder than most other people. The food police eye you suspiciously when you eat certain foods. Fear of complications hangs over your head. Sometimes it seems as if every time you see your doctor there's some new restriction or scary-sounding complication around the corner. Even when you have been dealing with all your new physical and mental changes, wham, your blood sugar readings go out of whack and leave you feeling rundown and fatigued. It's as if you are starting all over again from scratch.

This is part and parcel of having a chronic illness. Try to remember that having a chronic illness calls for a different way of looking at your health. It is no longer this static thing you can rely upon. You will have good days as well as bad days. And sometimes those bad days will last for a week or two or three. This unpredictability is to be expected. If it's any comfort, you are not alone. Over half the population of America has some kind of chronic health problem.

What do you do? How do you cope? For starters, check things out with your health network. Connect with family and friends and let them know what you need. Don't expect them to be able to read your mind and know that you want some TLC or need downtime. Tell them. You may need to cut back on your activities and social life for a bit. But you will be back in form soon. Load up on good books and funny movies. A hearty laugh can help you get over tough spots.

There's a great literary tradition surrounding illness. Typically, the illness jolts the hero or heroine into a new type of consciousness. They learn that they are not their illness, they are much more than that. In literature, there are a number of great illness novels, such as *The Magic Mountain*, by Thomas Mann, and *Mrs. Dalloway*, by Virginia Woolf.

FIRST PERSON INSIGHTS

The new, improved me

I was always suspicious of those stories about people who changed their lives around after they came down with some dire illness. But after my own prolonged bouts with diabetes, I can now appreciate those stories. Having diabetes has changed my spiritual understanding of myself and my place in the world. It has taken about four years to finally get my diabetes under control, and in those years, I've learned to let go of the little things. I had to—I was too tired to keep up appearances. I learned to "let go and let live." I call it my spiritual makeover.

—Sonya S., Philadelphia, PA

Helpful resources

The Chronic Illness Workbook
by Pat Fennel

Recrafting a Life
by Charlie Johnson and
Denise Webster

On Being Ill
by Virginia Woolf

Illness As Metaphor
by Susan Sontag

American Diabetes Association
www.diabetes.org
The ADA can help you find diabetes
support groups and offers a collection of books and other resources
for coping.

Pregnancy

Diabetes and pregnancy
planning for tight control

There's no reason a woman with diabetes can't be a mom. Yes, you will have to take extra care and work a bit harder, but you and your baby will be just fine. Still, diabetes can complicate matters, so it's best to talk with your doctor before becoming pregnant, because there are risks. For example, the risk of birth defects is increased in a diabetic pregnancy, yet with good control the risk can be brought very close to that of a nondiabetic pregnancy.

Depending on whether you have type 1, type 2, or gestational diabetes, your treatment plan during pregnancy will differ. Yet the advice you are likely to get from your obstetrician is the same: Good blood glucose control will help both mother and baby.

Part of the reason that good glucose control is important is that diabetic complications, such as eye, nerve, and kidney problems, can be brought on or worsen during pregnancy if blood sugar is not tightly controlled. However, these problems typically recede after the pregnancy and do not appear to increase the risk of developing complications later in life. Talk to your doctor about seeing an obstetrician who specializes in higher-risk pregnancies.

You should also see your diabetes doctor more often during the pregnancy. It's a good idea to see her once each week or every two weeks as things progress, depending on what you work out with your health team.

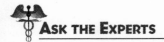

ASK THE EXPERTS

Can I breastfeed?

Yes, in fact it's a good idea. It's your choice, so talk to your doctor if you want to breastfeed. You might need to adjust your diet to increase the number of calories you take in, along the lines of what you ate during the pregnancy, to keep your sugar from dropping too low.

How do I keep my sugar up when morning sickness has me feeling nauseous all the time?

A fair question. A starch (crackers, melba toast) will help if you're feeling nauseated. Morning sickness is nausea when your stomach is empty, and it doesn't necessarily come only in the morning. A protein-and-carbohydrate snack at bedtime can help, too. One more tip: Drink between meals rather than at meals.

Is my baby at risk for developing diabetes?

According to the American Diabetes Association, a mother who has type 1 diabetes has a 1 in 15 risk that her baby will get diabetes. Interestingly, those numbers change with the mother's age. If the mother has the baby before the age of 25, the risk decreases to 1 in 100.

Gestational diabetes
dealing with insulin resistance

Some women develop a temporary form of diabetes, caused when hormones produced by the placenta during pregnancy reduce the effectiveness of insulin. This is called gestational diabetes, and it occurs during the growth (or gestation) of the baby in the womb. The condition usually disappears after delivery.

Who gets gestational diabetes? Between 3 and 6 percent of women develop the condition. There are certain factors that increase the risk of gestational diabetes. Women who are over 25, have a history of diabetes in the family, or are overweight have an increased risk of developing the disorder. Nonetheless, some women who have none of these risk factors develop gestational diabetes.

The diagnosis of gestational diabetes is usually made between 24 and 28 weeks into the pregnancy. This is why all pregnant women undergo a blood glucose test at that time. The diagnosis is made when:

◆ One hour after drinking a glucose drink, the blood sugar level is above 140 mg/dl. If blood glucose is above this level, a second test may be requested.

◆ In the second test, you are diagnosed with gestational diabetes if your blood sugar is found to meet two of the following criteria: The fasting blood sugar is above 105 mg/dl and after you drink a glucose drink, the blood glucose level is 190 mg/dl after 1 hour, 165 mg/dl after two hours, or 145 mg/dl after three hours.

As with other forms of diabetes, it's important to check your blood sugar often throughout the day. Tight control of gestational diabetes means working to keep blood sugar between 70 and 130 mg/dl. (These numbers are just an example. You doctor may suggest slightly different numbers depending on where you are in your pregnancy.)

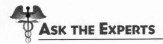

ASK THE EXPERTS

Do I have to take insulin?

Some women with gestational diabetes do need to take insulin. You will need to check your blood sugar often; if it isn't controlled by diet and exercise, insulin injections are necessary. If your blood sugar is above 100 mg/dl during a fasting glucose level check in the morning, or 120 mg/dl two hours after a meal, your doctor may prescribe insulin injections to protect the baby from increased glucose levels, which will cause him or her to gain excess weight.

How can I tell if my baby is healthy?

To check on the progress of your baby, there are a number of tests that can be performed at different stages of the pregnancy. A sonogram uses sound waves to visualize the fetus. This allows doctors to check its size and development. A non-stress test records the baby's heartbeat as the baby moves.

If I have gestational diabetes, what's my risk of developing type 2 diabetes after delivery?

The fact that your pancreas has difficulty overcoming the insulin resistance in pregnancy puts you at higher risk for developing diabetes later. The risk of developing type 2 diabetes within 15 years is about 50 percent higher if you have had gestational diabetes. So it's important to watch your weight and to exercise, which will greatly reduce your chances of getting diabetes later in life.

Pregnancy with type 1
taking extra care for a healthy pregnancy

Preparing for a baby requires a mother-to-be's attention to the details of diet and blood-sugar control, especially in the first trimester. A baby's organs are formed in the first six to eight weeks of pregnancy, so tight blood glucose control is crucial before pregnancy and early on in the pregnancy. Bringing your blood sugar consistently into the normal range will reduce the risk of birth defects to near that of mothers who don't have diabetes.

If you already have diabetic complications, such as kidney disease, cardiovascular disease, neuropathy, or uncontrolled high blood pressure, these conditions can worsen during pregnancy. This is very serious, and out-of-control diabetes can increase the risk of stroke or heart attack. You can minimize the risk of developing complications during pregnancy with an early thorough examination for any potential problems with your kidneys, eyes, and nerves (see pages 143–154 for more information).

Since hormones produced during pregnancy make insulin less effective, you will probably need to take more injections of insulin or go on an insulin pump. If you take ACE inhibitors, it's important to talk to your doctor before becoming pregnant, because these inhibitors can cause kidney defects in the baby.

If you're planning on getting pregnant, talk to your doctor first. While doctors no longer discourage women with type 1 diabetes from becoming pregnant, there's quite a bit of work to do to prepare for a safe pregnancy. Get a checkup and work to achieve very tight blood sugar control, ideally six months before getting pregnant. A checkup should include a glycated hemoglobin test, such as the hemoglobin A1c test. And work with a dietitian or doctor to determine how much weight you should gain.

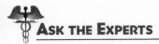

How often should I check my blood sugar?

You should check a lot more often than usual. Your doctor will encourage you to shoot for the tightest control of your life, testing seven times a day (probably before and after meals and at bedtime) or even more. Your doctor may also talk to you about daily ketone testing. Ketones are toxic substances given off when you burn fat for energy instead of glucose. You want your urine to be negative for ketones, as they can be harmful to both you and your baby.

What sort of exercise should I do?

Your health care team can help you find low-impact exercise that you will enjoy. Some concurrent conditions, such as high blood pressure, or problems with your eyes, kidneys, heart, or nerves, should be discussed with your doctor because some types of exercise can make these problems worse. Swimming and walking are good choices.

Any tips for a diabetic dad-to-be?

Try to keep stress at bay because anxiety can add to blood glucose volatility. Keep fast-acting sugar on hand, such as glucose tabs or tubes of cake frosting, which are a readily available choice for fast, portable sugar for low-blood-sugar moments. And watch out for sympathy cravings.

Pregnancy with type 2
adjusting the plan for mother and baby

If you have type 2 diabetes and become pregnant, the greatest change you are likely to see is in the way that you take your medicine. If you use diabetes pills, you will need to stop taking them, since they can pose a risk of birth defects. So if you don't already, you may need to start taking insulin injections (which have no impact on your developing baby). Injections can be a bit worrisome for some women, but it's important that you stop taking diabetes pills and still keep your blood sugar as close to the normal range as possible.

Insulin injections, along with increased blood sugar checking (seven or more times a day) can help you achieve the tight blood sugar control that's so important when you are pregnant. Doing so will reduce the risk of high blood pressure (hypertension), miscarriage, and birth defects. Extra glucose in the mother's blood can also cause the baby to grow too big, making the delivery harder for mother and baby.

Again, these risks can be greatly minimized by paying extra attention to blood glucose control. And there's good news. Studies show that pregnancy does not necessarily increase the mom's risk of diabetes-related complications over her lifetime.

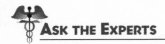

ASK THE EXPERTS

How much weight will I gain?

Your obstetrician will give you an idea of how much weight you should expect to gain, but 22 to 32 pounds is pretty typical. If you are under- or overweight before pregnancy, your doctor may advise more or less weight gain to be healthy.

When can I stop taking insulin shots?

You can usually stop taking injections shortly after delivery. After the baby is born, you will probably find that your blood sugar is easier to manage. However, breastfeeding can cause your blood sugar to drop, so it's a good idea to talk to your doctor or dietitian about adjusting your food intake to account for this. One more note: You should not take oral hypoglycemics if you are breastfeeding.

FIRST PERSON INSIGHTS

It's all in the testing

I seemed to be having quite a bit of trouble controlling my blood sugar during my pregnancy. My doctor recommended speaking with a dietitian. The dietitian showed me how to test for ketones daily. I also learned to increase my carbohydrate intake a bit when ketones were present to make sure I wasn't burning fat and passing ketones along to the baby (which can be harmful). I worked hard to get the best results I had ever had on my hemoglobin A_{1c} and found that my pregnancy went along easier than that of a nondiabetic friend of mine who was pregnant at the same time.

—Roxanne S., Telluride, CO

Helpful resources

Medline
www.nlm.nih.gov/medlineplus/
diabetesandpregnancy.html
Medline offers news and authoritative background information from
the National Library of Medicine, as
well as updated links to other useful
medical sites.

About.com
www.diabetes.about.com/cs/
gestationaldiab/
The About.com gestational diabetes
site connects you to advice on diabetes basics, nutrition during pregnancy, exercise programs for diabetic mothers, and treatment guidelines from around the Web.

Diabetic Gourmet
www.diabeticgourmet.com/
Healthy_Living/Diabetes_
and_Pregnancy
This site provides eating advice, of
course, but also offers helpful intro-
ductory information on diabetes
pregnancies, including articles on
weight gain, exercise programs, and
planning to become pregnant when
you have diabetes.

CHAPTER 13

Children with Diabetes

Stages of diabetes in children
what to expect

When children are first diagnosed with diabetes, there is often a short window of time, called the honeymoon period, when the body still produces insulin. This greatly reduces the need for insulin. Insulin injections are given during the honeymoon period, but the dose is typically quite small, perhaps just a few units a day. After the islet cells in the pancreas are no longer able to produce any insulin, the honeymoon period will end and diabetes care will become a bit more intense.

When kids are in their preteens, parents take care of most aspects of their diabetes, including testing for blood glucose, watching for low-blood-sugar episodes, and handling injections. One thing to remember is that tight control is not typically recommended for a child under 13. Your doctor and diabetes educator will help develop a treatment plan that is appropriate for the age of your child. Most kids, by the age of 12 or 13 (and some much earlier) are able to handle the majority of their diabetes care and will see the benefits, such as increased independence, of handling their injections and blood glucose control.

In the teenage years, young people face new temptations that may not fit perfectly with their health plan. While some variation from the health plan is predictable, it's important to recognize that the Diabetes Control and Complications Trial (DCCT) study showed how important tight control is in preventing and delaying diabetic complications.

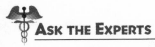

ASK THE EXPERTS

I'm concerned that my teenager is sometimes not testing his blood sugar, isn't paying attention to his diet, and cheats on results. What can I do?

In some cases a strict diabetes regimen enforced on a teenager may achieve the opposite result—the desire to rebel, to test limits, and perhaps to turn away from the treatment plan to feel more like a "regular" teen. This is understandable. If the situation becomes volatile and your child's care is obviously at risk, or has already caused serious incidents of hypoglycemia or hyperglycemia, consider talking to a counselor who has experience working with kids with diabetes.

How do I test my child's blood sugar at night?

Do a finger stick, the same as you do during the day. Also consider getting the latest development, a GlucoWatch. It measures blood sugar through the skin and will sound an alarm if blood sugar level goes above or below a given level (see page 210 for more information). You will still have to do two finger sticks each day to calibrate the watch. If blood sugar is a problem at night, give your child time-release carbohydrate bars which resemble granola bars. These snacks, eaten just before bed or before intense exercise, release 15 grams of carbohydrate over an eight-hour period.

Babysitter's tool kit

It's important to keep a glucagon shot in the fridge for serious hypoglycemic episodes that cause unconsciousness. Make sure that everyone (adults and older children) in the family (and your babysitter) know how to use it (see page 42 for more information).

After the diagnosis
adjustment and a little extra planning

If your child is diagnosed with diabetes, you will have plenty of questions: Can your child still play sports? What about sleepovers? Is camp safe? (The answers are yes, yes, and yes.) And those are just for starters. Many of the questions will depend on how old your child is when he or she is first diagnosed. And some of them—for instance, when is it time to hand over the responsibilities of diabetes management to your child?—will depend not only on the child's age but also on how well he or she adapts to the new situation. For many of your most urgent concerns, though, there are relatively straightforward answers.

Your doctor and diabetes educator (see pages 67–82) will help you tailor a health plan to your child. If you haven't already, you might also consider how your child might benefit from working with a pediatric endocrinologist, who specializes in dealing with kids with diseases that affect the endocrine system, such as diabetes. A pediatric endocrinologist has more experience working with diabetic children than your family doctor, a pediatrician, or an endocrinologist.

The time when your child takes on his or her own care depends on age and how ready you feel he or she is to handle the most important aspects of treatment. Even after your child starts managing his or her own treatment, you'll still want to oversee your child's diabetes.

A child with diabetes can do everything nondiabetic kids do, with a few adjustments and a little extra planning. When you talk to kids calmly and with confidence, they see that controlling their diabetes is a completely manageable situation. One in 600 kids has diabetes. So know that hundreds of thousands of children manage their diabetes successfully every day.

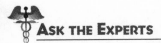 **ASK THE EXPERTS**

What should we tell the school?

Teachers and administrators should understand the effects of high and low blood sugar levels in a child with diabetes. The school nurse, or another trained adult, should be capable of helping your child with blood sugar testing, injections, or a glucagon shot if necessary. The school should also know that doctor's appointments and various sicknesses, which take a bit more time for individuals with diabetes to recover from, may require more absences from school than nondiabetic children need.

What activities can our child participate in?

Your child should be able to participate as other children do in classes, gym, sports, field trips, and other school and extracurricular activities. Sometimes your child will need access to fast-acting sugar, so the school should understand the need for your child to eat immediately when his or her blood sugar is low. Your child will also need to keep some fast-acting sugar on hand at all times. In some cases, children with diabetes need to excuse themselves to check blood sugar, and they should test for ketones (see pages 131–142) when blood sugar is over 240 mg/dl.

I'm that child
i've got diabetes. What now?

Being a kid is tough enough, but being diagnosed with a chronic disease will certainly add a bit more difficulty. There's a lot to deal with, but it won't stop you from making friends, eating well, and playing sports or any other activity you enjoy. You probably already know that you will watch your diet more carefully than other people do. You will also test your blood sugar and adjust the amount of insulin you take, based on how many carbohydrates you eat at a meal. You will need to keep candy or glucose tabs on you all the time for low-blood-sugar moments. And you will need to see a doctor several times a year.

The good news is that diabetes won't prevent you from doing anything you want—just take a look at two famous people, actress Halle Berry and Portland Trail Blazers center Chris Dudley. It didn't stop them, and it won't stop you. Will it make you different from other kids? Not really. Lots of children have diabetes, about 130,000 in the United States.

How will your friends react? Many of them will be curious about aspects of your diabetes. Pull out your blood glucose meter, and your nondiabetic classmates may even want to try it. And why not? Change the lancet and let them get a sense of how you take care of yourself. Your friends may even be impressed by the strength you show in taking injections, testing your sugar, and generally watching your meals a bit more carefully than they do.

It's completely understandable if you sometimes feel self-conscious, especially when you take medicine or check your sugar in public. Some children handle their shots and testing right in the open. Others are more discreet and head to a rest room to deal with their care. The bottom line? It's up to you. Do whatever makes you feel comfortable.

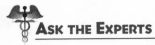

I'm 14 and I get embarrassed when my parents talk about my diabetes like I'm not even there. What can I do?

Let your folks know how you feel. Be honest without blaming them. They are used to taking care of you, so cut them some slack. Your parents will always care about how you take care of yourself, but eventually you will take charge of your diabetes care, with little or no help from your parents. They need to see that you can handle the challenges of your diabetes, one of which is talking about it. Learning how to talk about a chronic illness takes some practice (see pages 164–165 for pointers).

Sometimes my parents give me too hard a time about my diabetes control. Can't they understand that I just want to be a kid sometimes, and do the things other kids do?

If you feel that your parents are overprotective, it might be a good time to talk to a diabetes educator together. You could also speak with a therapist who has experience in diabetes care. Rigid rules are hard to follow and may lead to less compliance with your plan. And remember that there's power (and good diabetes control) in moderation.

What's in a candy?

When you need fast-acting sugar, sometimes a little candy can do the trick. But how much? You should use about 15 grams of carbohydrate to raise your blood sugar. Here are some common candies and the number it takes to have 15 grams of carbohydrate:

- 5 Lifesavers
- 15 pieces of candy corn
- 10 jelly beans
- 6 Hershey's Kisses

- 1 mini-pack of M&M's
- 4 Starbursts
- 15 Skittles

A family experience of illness
and a kitchen of friendly food

Diabetes is an illness that affects the way a family eats, works, and travels together. There will be adjustments, but they don't have to be earthshaking. Your family should not feel compelled to change old habits completely. But it does call for a healthy reassessment of how your family deals with food. To someone with diabetes, food is not just fuel or comfort—it is medicine.

Should you keep sugar-filled foods and snacks in the house? Children need to watch what they eat a bit more carefully now, but they can still eat the things they love in moderation. The important thing is to watch food intake carefully and take the appropriate amount of insulin to counteract the carbohydrates in meals and snacks.

That said, setting up a kitchen with foods that are friendly for someone with diabetes will create an environment that is healthy for the whole family. Everyone in your house will benefit from eating less refined sugar and fewer refined breads, focusing more on whole grains and fewer saturated fats, and watching caloric intake.

Some things, such as planning a meal or a trip, take a bit more time, so it's best to plan ahead. Get diabetic supplies beforehand so you won't have to rush after work to refill a prescription. You can also order supplies by mail. Often these mail-order houses handle automatic refills and bill your insurance company, so you don't need to make late-night trips to the pharmacy or disrupt a family gathering when your child informs you that the last bottle of insulin is empty.

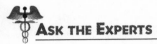

Will other children in the family resent the attention our child with diabetes receives?

Certainly this can be an issue. An open discussion with the children is usually a safe bet. Siblings can feel left out when so much attention is focused on one child. Explain that you care just as much for all your children, whether they have diabetes or not. Joining a support group or going to a family counselor can be a good way for all members of your family to feel included.

Our kids seem very worried about their sibling who has type 1— what should we tell them?

Answer their questions about diabetes (or seek out the answers together) and encourage them to let you know when they're worried. Tell them that long-term health problems related to diabetes are not inevitable. You may find that simply talking about their fears can help allay them to some degree.

My husband wants to go out, but I am afraid to leave our eight-year-old son with a sitter. What can I do?

It's easy to become overwhelmed as parents of a child with diabetes. But you do need to get out and spend time alone with your spouse. If you cannot find a family member to babysit, then identify a capable sitter and train her how to give insulin injections and check blood sugar. The sitter should have access to your doctor's or diabetes educator's phone contact information in case of an emergency. In case of a hypoglycemic attack, when your child cannot eat or drink something with sugar in it, the sitter should also know how to administer a glucagon shot.

Activities for children
all you need is some extra planning

With encouragement, children with diabetes can learn to be independent and confident about controlling their diabetes. The lessons they learn about managing their diabetes are valuable life lessons, too. As a parent, your goal is to guide and empower and then learn how to let go. This can be a challenge, especially when children enter adolescence, a stage often marked by defiance.

One big rite of passage for all children is their first sleepover. When your child is emotionally ready to spend the night at a friend's, here are some tips:

◆ Bring contact numbers for you and your child's physician. Explain your child's condition to the friend's parents.

◆ Put fast-acting sugar in his or her backpack. About five Lifesavers will do the trick if your child doesn't want to carry glucose tablets. Glucose tablets are often a good choice, though, and are unlikely to be snacked on by pals.

◆ Have your child test blood sugar before bedtime. A snack of carbohydrate and protein can help ward off lows in the night.

◆ Have your child wear a MedicAlert bracelet or other identification in case of emergency. Another possibility for young children is a temporary diabetes tattoo, available from a company called DiBon Systems (see Helpful Resources on page 202).

◆ Pack ketone testing strips for when blood sugar is over 240 mg/dl.

Children with diabetes are certainly capable of participating in all the usual sports, dances, and other strenuous activities. Again, all that your child needs is a little heads-up about activities so he or she can prepare. Let the coach or leader know that your child is diabetic and might need to check blood sugar and have a quick snack if necessary.

Diabetes camp

Often children who are feeling different or isolated because of their diabetes can benefit by joining in activities with other children with diabetes. Engaging in camp activities with other kids with diabetes can make your child's situation seem more routine and easier to manage. Camps, such as those listed on the American Diabetes Association Web site (**www.diabetes.org**), offer knowledgeable doctors and nurses and, often, counselors who have diabetes. Other than canoeing and sports, what else will your child learn? Handling injections safely and with less pain, portion control of food, and carbohydrate counting. They will also do all the normal kid stuff, such as competitive and team-building games like hiking or swimming, besides taking classes in diabetes care.

FIRST PERSON INSIGHTS

His first time away from us

Our son, diagnosed at seven, became deeply worried at the thought of diabetic complications and how they might affect his ability to lead a normal life. To some degree we shared these worries, but our son was capable of handling most of his care by the age of 10. He took all his own shots, measured his blood sugar, and kept a log of his blood sugar results for when he met with his doctor. He seemed to have a good handle on his own care and, we thought, an excellent chance of coping well with diabetes. A trip to a two-week diabetes camp, despite his initial hesitation to go, seemed to buoy his spirits, especially when he realized how many other kids were in the same situation. A talk at the camp, given by a man who had been a diabetic since before insulin was available (80 years!), showed him that he could lead a full, healthy life. He was eager to sign up for next year's camp—no nudging necessary this time around.

—Randal K, Birmingham, AL

Helpful resources

*Guide to Raising a Child with
Diabetes*
by Linda Siminerios and Jean
Betchart

*Getting the Most Out of Diabetes
Camp: A Guide for Parents and Kids*
American Diabetes Association

Sticking . . . but not Stuck
A newsletter published by Callie
Cox, a teenager with diabetes. The
publication also solicits contribu-
tions from kids. A one-year subscription is $15. Callie Cox, 115
North Meadows Place, Jackson, MS
39211

**The Juvenile Diabetes Research
Foundation**
Kids Online offers news, tips, and
information on diabetes self-care.
www.jdrf.org/kids

Children with Diabetes
www.childrenwithdiabetes.com
This often updated site is a great
starting place. It offers information
for those starting out as well as
advice on kid-specific health care.
Started by the parents of a child
with type 1 diabetes, this excellent
site covers a range of topics and
offers reviews of meters and other
products from a diabetic kid's per-
spective.

Reality Check
www.realitycheck.org.au
Out of Australia comes this site,
written by and for kids and young
adults. The site goes light on medical terminology and heavy on anecdotal information, a nice counter-
point to the authoritative, if dry,
information available elsewhere on
the Web.

DiBon Systems
Sells temporary diabetes identification tattoos, developed by diabetes
educators for kids.
www.dibonsystems.com

Cutting-edge Research

Living history
closing in on what causes diabetes

Diabetes has been around for centuries. The first-century Greek physician Arateus gave diabetes its name, but hundreds of years passed before anyone knew what caused diabetes or how to treat it.

Because physicians knew the condition caused sugar to spill into the urine, diabetes was officially diagnosed in the 11th century by tasting the urine. Diabetes was also diagnosed by pouring the urine of a patient near an anthill; it would attract the ants and provide a diagnosis. Chemical tests that could detect the presence of sugar in urine were developed in the 19th century.

It wasn't until 1922 that the hormone insulin was discovered by Frederick G. Banting. This discovery turned diabetes from a fatal disease to a treatable one. The young surgeon worked with another researcher, Charles H. Best, and a biochemist named James B. Collip to purify insulin and administer it to dogs that had had their pancreases removed. Banting and Best were able to develop a form of insulin that worked in humans. Along with J.J.R. Macleod, a physiologist at the University of Toronto, Banting was awarded the Nobel Prize in Medicine in 1923. (Before insulin was discovered, the only way to keep people with diabetes alive was to put them on a strict regimen of exercise and essentially a starvation diet. Even those who maintained this miserable treatment lived for only a year or two.)

The history of diabetes is still unfolding. In 1987 researchers determined that most people with type 1 diabetes have certain antibodies that identify islet cells to be destroyed by the body's immune system. This discovery helps clarify what causes diabetes, but it's still unclear why the antibodies begin marking these cells as foreign. The 1990s saw a flurry of diabetes research, including two groundbreaking studies that connected tight control of diabetes with a dramatic reduction in the risk of diabetic complications for individuals with both type 1 and type 2 diabetes.

Red-Letter Dates in Diabetes History

The history of insulin is actually quite short. Until a little over 80 years ago, there was no effective treatment for diabetes. People who had the disease died in a year or two at the most. The discovery of insulin and the means to inject it into people whose pancreases no longer produce the hormone earned its discoverers the Nobel Prize in 1923. Here's a quick look at some important dates in insulin history:

1901 Physician Eugene Opie discovers that the pancreatic beta cells produce a substance that prevents diabetes. It will be another 20 years before the substance is identified as insulin and used to treat patients.

1921 Insulin is extracted, and made ready for injection, by Frederick G. Banting, Charles H. Best, James B. Collip, and J.J.R. Macleod.

1922 Insulin injection is first used as a treatment for diabetes. The first patient is 14-year-old Leonard Thompson.

1966 Surgeons perform the first pancreas transplant at the University of Minnesota.

1983 The first synthetic human insulin is introduced.

1993 The Diabetes Control and Complications Trial (DCCT) reports that tight control of type 1 diabetes through frequent testing and adjustment of insulin can delay or prevent complications of diabetes, and delay their progression if they have already started.

2000 In the summer, Canadian researchers successfully perform islet transplants in several patients. The long-term effects of the transplants are unknown, but they look promising. Clinics around the country are now transplanting insulin-creating islet cells using this method, called the Edmonton Protocol.

The transplant cure
success comes with side effects

Diabetes is often the result of a malfunctioning pancreas. This makes its cure elegantly simple: a pancreas transplant. The first one was done in 1966 at the University of Minnesota. Since then, thousands of people with diabetes have received transplants, often when a transplanted kidney is also necessary.

So why doesn't every person with diabetes get a pancreas transplant? Because every transplant requires the patient to take antirejection drugs for life. These drugs suppress the immune system so it will not reject the transplanted pancreas. And because antirejection drugs suppress the immune system, they increase the risk of contracting common illnesses, including bacterial and viral infections. They can also increase the risk for certain types of cancer. These side effects can be daunting to people who are too ill from their diabetes to tolerate the side effects of a transplant.

Another possibility is to transplant new insulin-producing islet cells onto a malfunctioning pancreas. Islet transplantation is still in the clinical-trial stages, but the results are impressive. The insertion of insulin-producing islets, which make up just 1 percent of the pancreas, is a painless procedure that takes less than an hour. Like a pancreas recipient, an islet-cell recipient starts making insulin once the treatment is complete. However, islet recipients (like pancreas recipients) also need to take immunosuppressant drugs for life.

Another drawback to islet or pancreas transplantation is the lack of donors. There are more than a million people with type 1 diabetes in the United States, but fewer than 6,000 pancreases are donated each year. Some researchers are experimenting with the idea of using islets from pigs, which could provide an endless supply. But further study is needed, and the limited supply of human islets will continue to be a hurdle to this much anticipated method of curing diabetes.

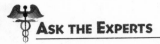
Who gets pancreas transplants?

Most of the people who receive pancreas transplants have developed a serious condition known as **hypoglycemic unawareness.** After years of living with diabetes, these people cannot seem to sense when their blood sugar levels are dangerously low. That's because they often do not experience the common physical signs of low blood sugar, such as nervousness, shakiness, light-headedness, and profuse sweating. (The only treatment solution is constant monitoring of glucose levels.) Other transplant recipients have at least one serious diabetic complication, such as kidney disease or eye disease. Currently, only a handful of people have received islet transplants in clinical studies.

How can I find information about islet transplantation?

The Islet Trials Web site (**www.isletservice.org**) provides loads of up-to-date information on islet transplantation. It even hosts online chats about transplantation with leading doctors and researchers from around the country. The site also provides a directory of transplant centers that you can use to find the islet transplant center nearest to your home and contact that center directly.

FIRST PERSON INSIGHTS

Hypoglycemic blues

After years of having diabetes with little problem, I suddenly had difficulty sensing when my sugar was low. I was running a bit late to meet my husband one afternoon when I passed out just as I got up to leave my office. Later, I got on the Web and researched hypoglycemic unawareness. Now I test my blood sugar more frequently to ward off lows. And I always test before driving. I've registered with an islet transplant study at the university hospital near my home, and I'm hopeful that someday an islet transplant will make my hypoglycemic incidents a thing of the past.

—Sharon L., St. Paul, MN

Improved testing and delivery
simpler, easier, and pain-free ways to test

In 2015 a young child diagnosed with diabetes may be given an outpatient treatment, handed a lollipop, and sent home, diabetes-free. Today glucose testing and insulin shots are still the norm. While a cure isn't right around the corner, researchers have done much to improve treatment. So, what advances can we expect to see in the near future?

◆ It's likely that an insulin pump, which delivers insulin continuously over the day and short bursts of insulin at mealtime, will be connected to a sensor implanted under the skin that can detect blood glucose levels, essentially creating an artificial pancreas for people with type 1 diabetes.

◆ Researchers and physicians will continue to improve techniques for insulin-producing islet transplants.

◆ Insulin taken by a means other than injection, such as with an inhaler or in pill form, could be widely used.

Research for a cure for type 2 diabetes is more complicated. Finding a replacement for the pancreas won't do the trick. Most people with type 2 diabetes have insulin resistance, in which the body cannot properly use the insulin made by the pancreas. If the pancreas fails, replacing it won't help.

In the meantime, researchers are developing better ways to treat diabetes. Methods of testing blood sugar that don't involve painful finger sticks have been under development for some time. And today a watchlike device is available that can test your blood sugar three times an hour without pricking your finger. We will continue to see improvements in diabetes care that will make the disease simpler to deal with.

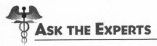
The doctor says my overweight husband is at high risk for developing type 2 diabetes. What should he do to prevent getting it?

Because obesity is strongly correlated with type 2 diabetes, he should lose weight. It is important that he eat a low-calorie, well-balanced diet that contains all the necessary nutrients his body needs (see pages 84–87). He also needs to exercise. There is a correlation between a sedentary lifestyle and diabetes. See pages 38–39 for more on the value of exercise.

FIRST PERSON INSIGHTS

How I became an advocate for diabetes

After I was diagnosed with type 2 diabetes, I headed for the library and read everything I could find on it. I came across the monthly magazines published by the American Diabetes Association and the Juvenile Diabetes Research Foundation. They have articles that focus on taking care of your diabetes and breakthroughs in research. The JDRF's magazine is called *Countdown*, and the ADA's magazine is *Forecast*. The more I read, the more interested I got. The next thing I knew, I picked up the phone and called the American Diabetes Association (800-342-2383) and asked how I could help. They got me in touch with their volunteer office. Because I had done so much reading, they asked me to help answer their hotlines in our local city chapter. I was delighted. It was wonderful talking to others with the same problem and sharing information with them.

—Sally R., Scottsdale, AZ

Less painful testing
every 10 minutes without drawing blood

Most people with diabetes have a love-hate relationship with their glucose meter. The very sharp, Tic-tac–size metal lancets that are used to draw the blood sample hurt. Yet studies have clearly shown how important it is to check blood sugar to keep your glucose in the normal range and prevent, or delay, complications. Thankfully, a number of new, less painful or pain-free testing methods are available or in development.

One painless meter, called the GlucoWatch Biographer, is now available. The Biographer is a testing device that measures your blood glucose every 10 minutes, without drawing blood. This meter applies a small electrical current that pulls glucose from the skin. You can set the watch to alert you if the reading is higher or lower than a level you're comfortable with.

The watch is a bit large, more like a slim pack of cards than a watch, really, but it can be very useful, especially if you have low blood sugar in the night, when you might not recognize the symptoms. The technology is new, and the cost is high (about $2,400, or six times what a regular glucose meter costs). As the price comes down and the technology improves, the GlucoWatch could be quite helpful. It's still a companion to, not a replacement for, testing with a regular glucose meter. If you think the GlucoWatch might be good for you, talk to your diabetes educator or physician and ask about other patients' experiences with it. Then check with your heath insurer; quite a few cover some of the cost.

MiniMed, which also makes insulin pumps, sells the Medtronic CGMS (continuous glucose monitoring system), an implantable meter that measures blood glucose many times over several days. A doctor can download the readings of the meter to a computer to look for blood sugar trends over several days, and then make adjustments to help you get your blood glucose levels where they should be.

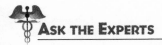

My fingers are sore from testing my blood sugar. Are there any glucose tests that don't just test the fingers?

Devices that use very small drops of blood to measure glucose are now widely available; some of them allow you to draw blood from the upper arm or forearm and are nearly painless. Not all can be used in alternative sites such as these, so it's important to read the packaging or ask a pharmacist before you buy one. The Therasense Freestyle and the One-Touch Ultra are two commonly used glucose meters that allow you to test with a small blood sample drawn from areas other than your fingers.

I've heard about a device that measures blood sugar using infrared light. How can I get one? And how much do they cost?

Another possible painless glucose meter could use an infrared beam of light, passed through a finger, to measure glucose in the blood. Sound futuristic? It is. Infrared testing has been discussed and studied for years, but the device is not yet available. A number of companies have claimed to produce infrared glucose-testing devices. However, these were very expensive, costing many thousands of dollars, and they did not prove to be effective. The Food and Drug Administration has forced several of them off the market.

How can I take part in a clinical trial of a new glucose-testing device?

Talk to your diabetes-care team, including your doctor, dietitian, or diabetes educator. They should be aware of clinical trials that might be taking place near your home. If they are not aware of any trials you may be interested in, they should be able to put you in touch with someone who might know more. Be sure to give them a chance to determine whether the trial could be useful to you and, more important, whether it's safe for you.

Insulin improvements
new insulin pills and inhalers

Researchers are working on making existing treatments for diabetes more efficient, less painful, and, in the case of insulin, easier to take. In the United States, about 4 million people with type 1 and type 2 diabetes inject insulin daily, according to the Centers for Disease Control. So a less painful way of delivering insulin could be an attractive alternative to injections for millions of people, who spend billions of dollars on insulin every year. Imagine insulin that's as easy to take as an aspirin.

The catch? Insulin, if taken orally, is digested by enzymes in the stomach. So how can you take insulin by mouth without its being digested in the stomach? Several new types of insulin, in a specially protected pill form or an inhaler form, are being tested.

- ◆ Insulin delivered as a pill is one pain-free alternative. One pill under development slips insulin past the stomach and into the small intestine where it breaks down and is then absorbed into the bloodstream. It is in clinical trials.

- ◆ A dry, very fine powdered insulin delivered via an inhaler device, similar to that used by people with asthma, is currently in clinical trials. The insulin is absorbed through the lungs. Another inhalable insulin type is a liquid spray, like a mist, that is absorbed in the mouth before it reaches the bloodstream.

These orally administered insulins act quickly and are taken at mealtimes. Because the insulin is fast-acting, it would not replace the need for injections entirely. Those who take oral or inhaled insulin will still need a slow-acting insulin, such as glargine (Lantus). See page 33 for more information on insulin types.

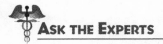

ASK THE EXPERTS

How can I get inhalable insulin?

Inhalable insulin is still under development but has been used in human trials and appears to work. The side effects on the mouth and lungs over a long period are not yet clear, so some experts recommend a wait-and-see attitude. Side effects might include a persistent cough and slightly decreased lung capacity. You've only got two lungs, so experts suggest that patience may be in order. Smokers are also unlikely candidates for inhaled insulin.

Is there any way to avoid the pain of injections?

If you take insulin and the pain is a primary concern, you might consider using an insulin pump, which requires insertion of the delivery cannula every two to three days, rather than syringes to inject insulin several times a day.

When will insulin pills be available?

Insulin in pill form is a promising advance, yet there will be at least several more years of testing before insulin pills are widely available. The side effects, if any, are not yet known.

Helpful resources

*The American Diabetes Association
Complete Guide to Diabetes*
by Bruce Zimmerman and
Elizabeth A. Walker

GlucoWatch
www.glucowatch.com/us

Rick Mendosa is a well-known diabetes journalist who frequently
posts new findings and reports on
his Web site.
www.mendosa.com/diabetes.htm

DCCT Information
You can find information about the
1993 Diabetes Care and
Complications Trial at the National
Institute of Diabetes and Digestive
and Kidney Diseases.
www.niddk.nih.gov/health/
diabetes/pubs/dcct1/dcct.htm

UKPDS
United Kingdom Prospective
Diabetes Study
A study that shows that tight glu-
cose control is good for people with
type 2 diabetes, too.

Glossary

Adult onset diabetes See type 2 diabetes.

Alpha cell A cell that makes a hormone called glucagon which raises blood sugar. Alpha cells, like beta and delta cells, are found in the islets of Langerhans.

Alpha-glucosidase inhibitor A type of oral hypoglycemic that helps slow or halt the breakdown of starches and sugars.

Americans with Disabilities Act A law passed in 1990 that protects civilian employees who work for companies with more than 15 people. The law prohibits employers from asking potential employees whether they have diabetes.

Antibodies Proteins that protect the body from foreign substances. In type 1 diabetes, the body creates antibodies that attack the insulin-producing cells in the pancreas.

Aspart A very fast-acting insulin sold as Novolog. (See Lispro.)

Aspartame An artificial sweetener, often sold under the name NutraSweet.

Basal dose A small, continuous flow of insulin. Often refers to the basal dose from an insulin pump.

Beta cell A type of cell that makes the hormone insulin.

Biguanides A class of oral hypoglycemic that reduces the amount of glucose released by the liver, helping to keep blood sugar lower.

Blood glucose A simple sugar carried though the blood and used for energy. The body converts carbohydrates you eat into glucose.

Blood pressure The pressure of blood on the walls of the arteries.

Blood sugar (See Blood glucose)

Bolus A fast-acting dose of insulin, delivered to cover meals. Often used in reference to the bolus dose of an insulin pump.

Brittle A term used to describe diabetes that is marked by severe high and low blood sugar. Sometimes called labile.

Cannula When you have an insulin pump, you must insert a catheter, called a cannula, every few days, which passes the insulin through your stomach.

Carbohydrate An organic compound containing carbon, hydrogen, and oxygen atoms. In your body, carbohydrates are converted to sugar and absorbed into the bloodstream. Starches, sugars, vegetables, fruits, and dairy products contain carbohydrates.

Creatinine A waste product of protein, which is removed from the blood by the kidneys.

Creatinine clearance A test that measures kidney function. If creatinine clearance is low, and the level of creatinine is high, it's an indication that kidney function is impaired.

Delta cell A type of cell, found in the islets of Langerhans, that is believed to help regulate the production of insulin and glucagon.

Diabetes Control and Complications Trial (DCCT) A 10-year study of type 1 diabetics, completed in 1993, that showed that tight blood glucose control was significant in preventing and delaying diabetic complications.

Diabetes educator A nurse practitioner, dietitian, or other health professional who specializes in working with diabetic patients. Your doctor can help you find a diabetes educator if you think you'd like to meet with one.

Diabetes mellitus A disease marked by a higher than normal level of glucose in the blood. See type 1 diabetes and type 2 diabetes.

Diabetes pills (See Oral hypo-glycemics.)

Diabetic complications Short-term diabetic complications include hypoglycemia (low blood sugar) and hyperglycemia (high blood sugar). Long-term hyperglycemia can lead to more serious problems, such as eye, kidney, nerve, and cardiovascular disease.

Diabetic ketoacidosis (DKA) A medical emergency that occurs from a combination of high blood sugar and a lack of insulin, when the body begins to break down fat for energy. Ketones are produced when the body breaks down fat, and if insulin does not remove ketones from the blood, it can be very dangerous. DKA is treated with fluids and insulin, but if not treated immediately, it can lead to coma and can be fatal.

Diabetologist A physician who specializes in diabetes.

Endocrinologist A doctor who specializes in diseases of the endocrine glands, such as diabetes.

Fasting blood glucose A blood sugar test taken after a person has not eaten for 8 to 12 hours, usually in the morning. The test is used to diagnose diabetes as well as monitor the care of people who have diabetes.

Flu The flu, or influenza, is a respiratory infection. Common symptoms are aches, fever, headache, exhaustion, and a cough that lasts a week or more. The flu is about six times more likely to send you to the hospital if you have diabetes.

Gestational diabetes Some women develop a temporary form of diabetes, caused when hormones produced by the placenta during pregnancy reduce the effectiveness of insulin. Gestational diabetes appears during the growth of the baby in the womb. The condition usually disappears after delivery.

Glargine A relatively new insulin (sold as Lantus) that starts working one to two hours after injection, does not have a pronounced peak, and acts over 24 hours.

Glucagon Glucagon is a hormone produced in the pancreas by alpha cells. Your doctor can prescribe a shot preloaded with glucagon that, after injection, will make your liver dump stored glucose into your bloodstream. This will make your sugar rise quickly. The glucagon shot is injected like an insulin shot.

Glucose meter A device about the size of a pager or billfold, that tells you how much glucose is in your blood. To use the meter, you prick your finger and place a small drop of blood on a testing strip.

Glucose tablets Candylike chewable tablets used to treat hypoglycemia.

Glycemic index (GI) The glycemic index is a measurement that determines how quickly carbohydrates are converted to glucose. Lower-GI foods produce less of a spike in your blood sugar.

Glycosuria A condition caused when the blood glucose level is higher than normal, causing sugar to spill into the urine. Glycosuria usually happens at about 180 mg/dl or more.

Glycolated hemoglobin A_{1c} A test which measures glucose levels over 60 to 90 days. Glucose binds to hemoglobin molecules in your red blood cells. A red blood cell has a life of about 90 days. So, using a hemoglobin A_{1c} test, a lab can measure the average glucose in the blood over two to three months.

Honeymoon period When children are first diagnosed with diabetes, there is often a short window, called the honeymoon period, when the body still produces insulin. This greatly reduces the need for insulin, and it typically lasts for only a short time.

Hyperglycemia High blood glucose. Hyperglycemia can make you feel tired, sluggish, thirsty. Over the long term, hyperglycemia leads to serious diabetic complications.

Hypoglycemia. Low blood sugar, typically below 70 mg/dl. Sometimes called an insulin reaction, hypoglycemia can cause nervousness, shakiness, and extreme sweating and hunger, among other symptoms. Hypoglycemia is treated with fast-acting, carbohydrate-rich foods, such as glucose tablets or regular soda. Hypoglycemia can also be treated with a glucagon shot if the reaction is serious enough to cause unconsciousness.

Hypertension High blood pressure, which leads to increased risk of kidney damage, heart attack, and stroke.

Insulin Insulin is a hormone, produced by the pancreas, that helps the body use sugar for energy.

Insulin dependent diabetes mellitus (IDDM) (See type 1 diabetes.)

Insulin pump About the size of a pager, an insulin pump provides a small, continuous dose of insulin, as the pancreas does. The pump is a small, battery-operated machine connected to a vial (reservoir) of insulin. Insulin pumps deliver two different doses of fast-acting insulin, at different times. (See Basal dose and Bolus.)

Insulin resistance A condition in which cells cannot efficiently use insulin.

Islet Also called the islets of Langerhans, these bundles of cells found in the pancreas contain beta cells (which make the hormone insulin) and alpha cells (which make the hormone glucagon, which raises blood sugar).

Islet cell antibody test A test which can detect the presence of the antibodies that destroy insulin-producing beta cells.

Islets of Langerhans (See Islets.)

Juvenile diabetes (See type 1 diabetes.)

Ketones A byproduct created when your body begins to burn fat for energy. If your sugar gets very high, or when there's not enough food in your body for energy, ketones can build up in your bloodstream and spill into the urine. It's important to check for ketones, especially when you are sick, by using a urine sample and ketone testing strips (which are inexpensive and available at your pharmacy), when your blood sugar rises above 240 mg/dl.

Kidney disease Diabetics are at a higher risk for developing kidney (or renal) disease, which reduces the ability of the kidneys to filter the blood. In end-stage kidney disease, the kidneys fail permanently and dialysis is required.

Kidneys The kidneys (you have two) clean waste products and toxins from the blood.

Lente An intermediate-acting insulin that begins working in 2 to 6 hours, peaks between 4 and 14 hours, and lasts 18 to 24 hours.

Lispro The fastest-acting insulins you can purchase are called lispro, sold under the brand name Humalog, and insulin aspart, sold as Novolog. These insulins start working about 15 minutes after you take them. Aspart and lispro peak between 30 and 90 minutes after injection.

MedicAlert A nonprofit organization that sells bracelets and pendants that identify the wearer as having a medical condition. The bracelet can tell an emergency responder that you are a diabetic and provides a toll-free phone number to call. When contacted, MedicAlert sends the responding emergency team your medical history.

Meglitinides A class of oral hypo-glycemics that stimulate the pancreas to make more insulin, examples: Repaglinide (Prandin) and Nateglinide (Starlix).

Microalbuminuria Small amounts of protein in the urine.

Microaneurysm A small swelling of the retinal blood vessels that people who have had diabetes for years some-times get.

Neonatologist A doctor who focuses on the treatment of newborn babies.

Nephrologist A doctor who specializes in treating people with kidney dis-ease.

Nephropathy Kidney disease.

Neuropathy Nerve damage.

Noninsulin-dependent diabetes melli-tus (NIDDM) (See type 2 diabetes.)

Nonproliferative retinopathy A rela-tively common condition for people who have had diabetes for many years. In this form of retinopathy, capillaries expand and form pouches that are visible during an eye exam. It does not require treatment.

NPH An intermediate-acting insulin, also called N, that begins working 1 to 2 hours after injection, peaks between 6 and 10, and lasts for 12 to 16 hours.

Ophthalmologist An eye doctor. You should see one once a year to be checked for signs of retinopathy.

Oral hypoglycemics Medicine you take to help control type 2 diabetes. Oral hypoglycemics help lower blood sugar levels. These include sulfonyl-ureas and meglitinides (see Sulfonylurea).

Pancreas A banana-shaped, fist-sized organ that sits behind your stomach and makes the hormones insulin, which lowers blood sugar, and glucagon, which forces cells to release or produce glucose (raising blood sugar). The pancreas also pro-duces enzymes that help with diges-tion.

Peripheral vascular disease A form of atherosclerosis characterized by blockages of blood flow in the arms, feet, and legs. It can cause pain and slow healing of foot sores.

Proliferative retinopathy When blood vessels are damaged from chronic hyperglycemia, this more serious condition can cause new blood ves-sels to grow in order to carry the blood. But these new blood vessels are weak and may leak blood into the eye, making vision cloudy. Without treatment, this can lead to blindness.

Proteinuria A condition in which there is too much protein in the urine, which can be a sign of kidney damage.

Regular insulin A fast-acting insulin, also called R, that begins lowering blood glucose within 30 minutes and peaks two to five hours later.

Retina The lining in the back of the eye that senses light.

Retinopathy (See Nonproliferative retinopathy and Proliferative retinopathy.)

Saccharin An artificial sweetener sold under the name Sweet'N Low.

Sucralose An artificial sweetener mar-keted as Splenda.

Sulfonylurea An oral hypoglycemic medicine for diabetes that stimulates the pancreas to make more insulin.

Support groups Meetings where people can share information and experi-ences and get support in a safe atmosphere. Support groups are often led by a therapist, nurse, social worker, or diabetes educator. The facilitator can be helpful in making sure members' concerns are addressed and that medical information is accurate.

Type 1 diabetes A disease in which the pancreas does not make insulin, so glucose cannot enter the cells to be used for energy. In type 1 diabetes, the immune system attacks insulin-producing beta cells in the pancreas. Type 1 diabetes is less frequently called insulin dependent diabetes or juvenile diabetes.

Type 2 diabetes A disease in which the body cannot produce enough insulin, or there is resistance to the insulin produced. In some cases, the pancreas creates more insulin than is needed, but insulin resistance won't allow the insulin to help get sugar into the cells to be used for energy. Type 2 is now less frequently called non-insulin dependent diabetes or adult-onset diabetes.

Thiazolidinedione An oral hypoglycemic that helps to reduce insulin resistance by increasing the sensitivity of the muscles to insulin.

Transcutaneous nerve stimulation A procedure sometimes used by patients with neuropathy. This electric stimulation, like acupuncture, is believed to promote the production of natural painkillers.

Triglyceride A type of fat in the blood. High levels of triglycerides can increase the risk of stroke and heart attack.

Index